Walking Isn't Everything

By Jean Denecke

First Edition

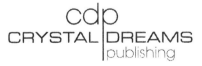

CRYSTAL DREAMS
publishing

Oshawa, Ontario

Walking Isn't Everything

by Jean Denecke

Managing Editor: Kevin Aguanno
Acquisitions Editor: Sarah Schwersenska
General Editors: Kristin Gruenewald and Keith Storey
Copy Editor: Susan Andres
Typesetting: Peggy LeTrent
Cover Design: Troy O'Brien

Published by: Crystal Dreams Publishing
(a division of Multi-Media Publications Inc.)
Box 58043, Rosslynn RPO, Oshawa, Ontario, Canada, L1J 8L6.

http://www.crystaldreamspublishing.com/

Paperback	ISBN-10: 1-59146-192-8	ISBN-13: 9781591461920
Adobe PDF ebook	ISBN-10: 1-59146-201-0	ISBN-13: 9781591462019
Microsoft LIT ebook	ISBN-10: 1-59146-202-9	ISBN-13: 9781591462026
Mobipocket PRC ebook	ISBN-10: 1-59146-203-7	ISBN-13: 9781591462033
Palm PDB ebook	ISBN-10: 1-59146-204-5	ISBN-13: 9781591462040

Published in Canada and the United States of America.

CIP data available from the publisher.

Table of Contents

Editorial Note

Jean Lucille Leeper Denecke contracted polio in 1946. Although she never regained the ability to walk, she was able to take care of some of her personal needs, write, dial a phone, and breathe without assistance. She was active in her church and charitable organizations, and in 1954, founded a small business, which she ran from her home by telephone. With assistance, and particularly support from her husband, she raised her family, ran her household, and was an inspiration to others.

Kristin Gruenewald (editor) is the daughter of Jean Denecke. She is a retired social worker and public administrator. She lives in Michigan with her husband Bob and dog Rudy. She appreciates her mother more each day that she lives.

Keith Storey (editor) is the nephew of Jean Denecke. He is currently a professor of education and Special Education Program Chair at Touro University in Vallejo, California. He served six years as a classroom teacher working with people with a variety of disability labels. His research interests include inclusion, supported employment, transition from school to adult life, and positive behavior supports. He lives in California with his wife, two children, two cats, and a dog.

Walking Isn't Everything

Dedications

Original Dedication From Jean Denecke

To Kris, her heritage.

Kris's Dedication

To Mom and Dad

Keith's Dedication

To my cousin Kris, who at a family reunion a couple of years ago, casually mentioned in passing "the book that my mother wrote about having polio." This was news to me, even though Kris, of course, has known of my professional career in the disability field. Kris got me started on genealogy and together we have researched our family history but for some reason, it did not occur to her that I would be interested in the book! But I thank her for sharing her mother's book with me and I am very honored to have helped in sharing it with other family members as well as the public (a mere fifty-six years after it was written). It has increased my understanding and appreciation of her parents who were both wonderful people (Kris too!)

Walking Isn't Everything

Foreword

Warm Springs — Yesterday and Today

Founded by Franklin Delano Roosevelt in 1927, over five years before he became president, the Georgia Warm Springs Foundation was a unique community in U.S. history. Even before it became world famous as a polio treatment center in the 1940s and 1950s, it was a place with a prevailing spirit all its own—a spirit of understanding, togetherness, hope, determination, and compassionate care.

"We were a family," one polio survivor, James Woods of Fillmore, Indiana, recently remarked, many years after he learned to walk again on the Warm Springs campus. And for most of the 125 or so polio patients who were being treated at Warm Springs at any one time, they were a second family in every sense of the word.

It was not that their primary families did not remain extremely important in all their lives—it was simply the fact that they shared a disease that had rendered them outcasts in a society that all too often did not deal with disabilities very

9

well. With their futures altered and their real-life families trying to cope and provide as best they could, they came to Warm Springs and bonded with peers from all over the country in a special way that marked them all as survivors, leading eventually to productive lives and careers.

They bonded not only among themselves but also with the staff of Warm Springs. In fact, while no one ever established for sure how the polio virus was transmitted, there was no doubt that life together at the Foundation transmitted the beforementioned spirit in such a way that no one who was treated or worked at the West Georgia facility could fail to catch what became known as "the spirit of Warm Springs."

Despite leaving home for difficult therapy and, in most cases, multiple operations spread over a number of years and visits, their Warm Springs family was always here waiting to receive them, ready to support and nurse them on their individual roads to recovery, and ready also to take their minds off the difficult hands they had been dealt. Wheelchair races, first loves, plays and presentations, endless childhood pranks, and even Founders Day dinners with the president were all part of the warm and caring atmosphere that pervaded this special and somewhat isolated community at the base of Pine Mountain.

Designed to resemble a college campus rather than a hospital, the camaraderie of college life was very evident despite the medical necessities that brought it into existence in the first place. Its historic Quadrangle and Schoolhouse, which kept the young patients from getting behind during extended stays, still bring to mind the University of Virginia and FDR would not have had it any other way.

Fine linen tablecloths and jacketed waiters were also the order of the day in the Georgia Hall Dining Room, as support for the facility increased with notoriety and the influence provided by its famous founder. Presidential birthday balls held throughout the country to raise money for the Foundation and polio research during FDR's twelve-plus years in office were forerunners of the March of Dimes after his death (April 12, 1945). The result was the race for "a cure" that was really no cure but a preventative—the Salk and Sabin vaccines that eventually eradicated future cases of the disease in this country during the 1950s and 1960s.

The impact of the vaccines influenced the way the facility did business, but not the spirit of the place. Gradually, the emphasis on polio shifted to persons with all types of disabilities, and along with the early therapists, who initiated "The Roosevelt Way," rehabilitation technology came to the forefront through the development of braces, crutches, and all kinds of individualized assistive devices. Warm Springs' pioneers in these fields would make their mark throughout the nation.

In 1964, the Foundation donated enough land to the state of Georgia to build the Georgia Rehabilitation Center, which stressed vocational rehabilitation for young people with disabilities, and in 1974, the state assumed management of the hospital as well, turning it all into the Roosevelt Warm Springs Institute for Rehabilitation, one of only nine state-managed rehabilitation centers in the country.

Today, eighty years after its founding, the Roosevelt Warm Springs Institute for Rehabilitation remains FDR's living legacy. With a stated mission of "empowering individuals with disabilities to achieve personal independence," it is truly a comprehensive rehab center specializing in both medical and vocational rehabilitation.

Approximately five thousand clients utilize Roosevelt Warm Springs' services each year, including students, usually ages 18–26, in the Vocational Rehabilitation Unit (VRU); inpatients in the Medical Unit for both long-term acute care and inpatient rehab; and outpatients from throughout the West Georgia area who will soon take advantage of brand new, 35,000-square-foot Blanchard Hall. Blanchard Hall is a one-stop shop for Roosevelt

Warm Springs Outpatient Services, including orthotics and prosthetics, seating and wheeled mobility, diabetic foot care, wound care, outpatient therapy, and outpatient physician care.

In addition, about six thousand people each year are guests at Roosevelt Warm Springs for professional conferences or disability camps at fully accessible Camp Dream, a 74-acre complex that along with the Frank C. Ruzycki Center for Therapeutic Recreation opened in the mid 1990s. Together, they provide unique recreation access to persons with disabilities in a state-of-the-art environment.

Young adults in the VRU with both learning and physical disabilities finish academic work and receive job skills. They are usually in residence about nine months while working on individualized programs designed to help them re-enter their local communities and the job force.

The Medical Unit is divided into two entirely separate inpatient hospitals—the Roosevelt Warm Springs Rehabilitation Hospital and the Roosevelt Warm Springs Long Term Acute Care Hospital. Each has its own staff and currently hosts up to thirty-two inpatients at a time. Roosevelt Warm Springs Outpatient Services offers clinics in the nearby towns of Newnan and LaGrange in addition to Warm Springs.

Except for state management, as opposed to private ownership, the culture remains much as it was during the polio era. Even as state employees for the last thirty-plus years, Roosevelt Warm Springs staff continue a rapport and feeling for the place that transcends decades. Some of them even still live on campus.

The entire 940-acre campus was designated a National Historic Landmark District in 1980 and it becomes more and more of an attraction (separate from FDR's Little White House State Historic Site) as the years go by. Although in need of renovation, the historic Quadrangle, Roosevelt Memorial

Chapel, and other buildings on campus, including the individual cottages that were here when FDR first purchased the property, all share in the unique story of the place—a story that people find inspiring and very much worth maintaining in the twenty-first century. Guided tours are offered twice daily and the HBO movie Warm Springs, which won numerous awards in 2005, is available at video rental stores nationwide.

The mineral-rich Warm Springs water that attracted Roosevelt in the first place still emerges at eighty-eight degrees and nearly nine hundred gallons per minute. In fact, every drop of water used on campus comes from the springs just as "the spirit of Warm Springs" that has not changed . . . and I hope never will.

Martin Harmon
Roosevelt Warm Springs
Public Relations Director

Walking Isn't Everything

Preface

Can you imagine yourself nonchalantly rolling down the sidewalk in a wheelchair, en route to a P.T.A. meeting at school? Well, I could not either, but that was five years ago before polio— before my wheelchair and I became one.

This is my story. It is a story I cannot tell medically or psychologically, but I can relate it as an intimate personal experience.

Physically, I am pretty much a mess. I cannot walk, lift my arms from the shoulder, turn myself over in bed, and my hands are far from normal. I spent eight months in an iron lung and even now, my breathing is just adequate and a severe cold could very well be fatal. I do not mean for this to sound pathetic. I have been subjected to some intense sympathy in the past five years, and it has always made me feel a little self-conscious, as though people must be talking about someone else because I just could not be that bad off.

Most polios who are left with extensive paralysis usually come to the point where suicide is their uppermost thought. I was no exception. I wanted my husband to bring rat poison to me at the hospital. Yet, approximately two years later, I was able to listen without batting an eye, or shedding a tear, when the staff doctor at the incomparable Georgia Warm Springs Foundation told me that no part of me had been undamaged by polio. I was able to listen while he outlined what, two years previously, would have seemed like meager improvements and to agree with him that I was lucky to be alive. By that time, my condition had become a relative thing, much like the man who was sorry for himself because he had no shoes, until he met a man without feet.

Today, except for my physical condition, I feel that I lead a perfectly normal life. I run my house through my housekeeper and my family. I do a bit of church work; I vote; I am a member of the troop committee of my daughter's Brownie organization; and if the weather permits, you will indeed see me with my family, wheeling to a school meeting.

In the past four years, there have been 132,000 persons stricken with polio. Of that number, only ten per cent are left crippled.

I hope that by telling my story I can help to convince those other polios and their families who are new to the battle that, no matter what the end result may be, it can well be worth the struggle with yourselves to try to return to normal living. I believe my family and I have won our battle just as surely, as if my physical recovery had been complete.

Introduction

What Is Polio?

Poliomyelitis is a viral disease and there are three types of poliovirus with different strains of each type. Poliovirus enters through the mouth and multiplies in the throat and gastrointestinal tract, then moves into the bloodstream and is carried to the central nervous system where it replicates and destroys the motor neuron cells. The destroyed cells are often the anterior horn cells of the spinal cord. These cells relay information that controls motor functions of the arms and legs and the destruction of these cells then leads to weakness of those limbs. The poliovirus can also infect neurons in the brainstem where breathing and swallowing are controlled. The symptoms of polio often started innocuously enough with a sore throat, stiff neck, sore muscles, fever, and/or headache, but then could very quickly develop into more severe conditions such as excruciating pain, paralysis, or even death. These individuals with a diagnosis of polio were often put very quickly into isolation wards in hospitals, often within hours of the diagnosis. In response to this need by individuals with breathing problems (only a small percentage of those with polio), the first mechanical respirator, or iron lung, was developed in 1929.

Polio was first defined as a specific disease entity in either the late seventeenth or late eighteenth century, depending upon different interpretations of the historical record. Michael Underwood provided the earliest known accurate description of polio in 1789. Polio occurred without distinction across class, gender, ethnic, and racial lines but more often in children than in adults. Polio became more common in the late nineteenth century, in part due to better efforts of cleanliness and sanitation that limited exposure to the virus and thus the ability for individuals to develop immunity. Approximately 1 to 3 percent of individuals infected with polio developed physical paralysis.

In the late nineteenth and early to mid-twentieth centuries, polio epidemics were common and they often resulted in panics in which people fled cities and other affected areas. For instance, in the summer of 1916, over fifty thousand children were sent out of New York City. Later in the summer, the opening of schools was postponed and police roadblocks were set up to keep people under the age of sixteen from entering the city. Between June and December of that year in New York City, there were 8,900 cases of polio and 2,400 deaths, which is a mortality rate of one in four for children.

The most famous person with polio was, of course, Franklin Roosevelt, the thirty-second president of the United States, who came down with polio in August of 1921 at the age of thirty-nine. Though openly acknowledging that he had polio, Roosevelt went to great lengths to hide the severity of his physical disability from the public, and there are only two known pictures of Roosevelt in his wheelchair. Roosevelt hid his disability by not using his wheelchair in public and appearing to be able to walk by holding himself up on one or two people walking next to him and swinging his legs. He also had many people walking with him in a group to make it difficult for people to see him clearly at these times.

In 1938, Franklin Roosevelt, his law partner Basil O'Connor, and others started the National Foundation for Control of Infantile Poliomyelitis (now known as the March of Dimes), which was dedicated to developing a vaccine to prevent polio. This effort was successful by 1955 with the successful inoculation in 1954 of nearly two million children who participated in the field trials by Dr. Jonas Salk and a team of researchers at the University of Pittsburgh.

In the 1940s, Sister Kenny, an Australian nurse, came to the U.S. and promoted a new treatment for polio that used warm compresses to relax painful and contracting muscles as well as massage and exercise for rehabilitation. This was in direct contrast to, and much more effective than, earlier efforts that involved immobilization of the damaged limbs with splints and body casts which resulted in further loss of muscles and movement.

At its peak in the United States in 1952, nearly fifty-eight thousand people became sick, twenty-one thousand were paralyzed, and over three thousand died from polio. By 1957, the number of cases of polio had fallen by 90 percent, and polio was eradicated in the United States in 1979.

A Personal Memoir—Contracting Polio in the Late 1940s

Jean Denecke's candid recollections about contracting the poliovirus in 1947 and the road she traveled to return to her life with husband Harry and young daughter Kris provide an intimate, even iconic, portrait of a polio survivor. Her story not only reflects experiences shared by thousands of children and young adults during a period in which polio epidemics ravaged communities throughout the United States, it also provides a glimpse of middle-class family and community life in post-World

Walking Isn't Everything

War II America and foreshadows the disability rights revolution that was to come.

Jean Denecke, a 28-year-old wife, mother, and homemaker when she became ill from the poliovirus, tells her story with one specific goal in mind—to inspire others to reclaim their lives after contracting polio. Her experiences and point of view take on broader meaning now, however, because they also are embedded in the historical framework of the polio epidemics of the early to mid-twentieth century. These epidemics spurred profound changes in medical research, philanthropy, and rehabilitation medicine and provided both leaders and foot soldiers for a new grassroots advocacy movement of people with disabilities and their supporters.

Poliomyelitis epidemics surged through U.S. cities during the early twentieth century. Throughout the 1940s and 1950s, the virus randomly assailed children and young adults primarily and generated widespread fear and terror. Characterized by fevers, malaise, headaches, joint and muscle pain, nausea, and for some, paralysis, polio struck nearly one hundred thousand people between 1952 and 1954 alone. In 1955, the Salk vaccine was shown in widespread trials to be effective in preventing the disease and an immunization program was launched. While polio has been eradicated in the U.S., estimates suggest that 600 thousand polio survivors are living in the country today, and the number worldwide could be tens of millions.

Behind these numbers, we find people such as Jean Denecke who never saw polio coming and never could have imagined how it would shape the direction of her life. Just as so many people who contracted polio in the 1940s and 1950s, she was thrown into a world she knew existed but one for which she and her family were not remotely prepared. Jean Denecke writes in clear, uncluttered prose about her first days in the hospital after contracting the poliovirus when she had little idea what was happening to her and less about what to expect. While the medical professionals around her understood the extent of polio's likely final impact on her capacity to walk, talk, breathe, and function, they conveyed little of that information to her. Furthermore, rigid hospital rules permitted family members only an ancillary role; they were generally consigned to visiting a half-hour a day if they lived nearby or an hour or two on occasional weekends if they lived at a distance. Recalling these early encounters, many polio survivors relate that the culture and practices surrounding care and treatment set the stage for months, if not years, of isolation from family, friends, school, jobs, and the common joys, challenges, and experiences of childhood and adult life.

While Jean Denecke's early days in the polio ward were fraught with pain and uncertainty, her recollection of the details of her care and treatment also begin to reveal a character and state of mind that, at its core, proved willful and determined. She was not only determined to break free of the hospital but also to shrug off the negative assumptions and limited expectations about her future life as a person with a disability that she knew were held by many around her. In 1947, people with disabilities, including people who had contracted polio, sparked pity, fear, and paternalistic attitudes. Principles of architectural accessibility, sophisticated assistive technology, and workplace accommodation that we now take for granted, were unheard of then. While veterans who had returned from WWII with significant disabilities were alive thanks to lifesaving medical advances, they and the government that represented them were just beginning to challenge physical and attitudinal barriers that prevented them from resuming their lives as civilians. In other words, there were no curb cuts so people who used wheelchairs could get around their communities or ramps into public buildings, shops, or restaurants. Technologic advances that are commonplace today, that were undeveloped then, include portable respirators so that people who needed them could even live outside of an iron lung and spend time in their community.

Walking Isn't Everything

Some public schools even had policies that barred admission of children with disabilities. They were either educated at home or attended segregated "disabled-only" schools.

Furthermore, a family such as Jean Denecke's had little access to practical help and support from community or government sources. The March of Dimes, founded in 1938 in response to the polio epidemics, funded the National Foundation for Infantile Paralysis that provided equipment such as wheelchairs and respirators, and later, in-home assistance. But at the time that Jean Denecke contracted polio, most families with a disabled member were required to manage and pay for caretaking, home modifications to accommodate a wheelchair user, transportation, and the like on their own. Jean Denecke's husband and parents—middle-class by the standards of the day—assumed most of the financial and personal responsibility for everything she needed after her release from the hospital, with the exception of devices provided by the National Foundation. If her family had been poor and/or also unable to care for her, she might have been forced to live in an institution for the balance of her life rather than return to her family home, regardless of her keen desire to resume her former life. In many respects, people experiencing significant physical and/or intellectual disabilities today are faced with the same choices.

For those who need significant supports that their family may be unable to provide or that may not be available in their community (such as personal assistance and supported living services), their only option is often to live in nursing homes or other institutional environments. According to the Centers for Disease Control, about 1.6 million people live in nursing facilities in the United States, including an estimated 30,027 persons with intellectual/developmental disabilities, based on 2005 estimates. In 2007, 10.7 million people with disabilities, age six and older, need personal assistance with one or more activities of daily living (such as taking a bath or shower) or instrumental activities

22

of daily living (such as using the telephone). This amounts to 4 percent of people in this age category.

Jean Denecke's account of her early treatment also reveals in palpable detail her experience with the Sister Elizabeth Kenny method of early rehabilitation. Until Kenny recognized the importance of early use of moist heat and stretching exercises to prevent polio-affected muscles from tightening, the prevailing treatment placed people in splints and immobilized them for weeks or months, causing wasting, contractures, and irreversible stiffness in some cases. Jean Denecke's forthright description of being treated with hot "packs" that were applied to her body several times during the day will resonate with most polio survivors as will her vivid description of living in an iron lung for many months. An iron lung is a device that assists breathing and looks like a large tube. The person whose breathing is being assisted lies supine in the tube with only his or her head exposed through a collar. Iconic in their own right, these items were staples of polio wards everywhere and numerous photos depicting them in use were displayed during 2005 at the groundbreaking exhibit on the history of polio mounted by the Smithsonian's National Museum of American History (now available on line at http://americanhistory.si.edu/polio/index.htm).

During a particularly difficult period, Jean Denecke forthrightly recalls feeling that her life was not worth living and that she considered suicide. She mentions that she even pleaded with her husband to help her with the suicide. Later, and in retrospect, she opines that many people who face the radical life-changing events that can be precipitated by contracting polio probably also considered ending their lives at some point. It has been documented that many newly injured or disabled people go through certain phases as they adapt to their altered situations that can sometimes include a period when they wish to end their lives, so Jean Denecke's experience fits within a familiar paradigm. It appears that she also reveals this moment deliberately to assure her intended readers that such a desire will pass and that one must not act precipitously. By turning this most personal and dramatic moment into a valuable life lesson, she has found an effective method that she calls upon frequently throughout the memoir to communicate to the audience her fundamental message of hope, optimism, and resiliency in the face of significant personal challenges.

It is interesting to note that Ed Roberts, who contracted polio at age fourteen, also wanted to commit suicide while in a hospital. Ed, too, changed his mind and went on to be the first person with a significant physical disability (he slept in an iron lung at night) to attend the University of California at Berkeley. He is widely credited with playing a leading role in founding the disability rights and went on to become one of the most prominent people in the disability rights independent living movement. Among his achievements are starting the first Center for Independent Living, starting the World Institute on Disability, and being the Director of the Department of Rehabilitation for the state of California.

When she first arrived at home after experiencing both the rigors and security of hospital life, Jean Denecke squarely faced the reality of her changed body and limited functional capacity. She had convinced her husband that she was ready to tackle the transition and should be allowed to come home because she missed her young daughter and desperately wished to resume her role as parent, wife, and homemaker. The long transition back to the world involved developing strategies to cope with significant paralysis that impaired her breathing, limited the use of her arms and hands, and required that she use a wheelchair for mobility and arm slings that allowed the use of her hands.

Jean Denecke's account of this transition, a process that took place over several years, illustrates the critical role of family and friends and, in particular, the stalwart commitment of her husband. He not only supported the family financially but also helped run the household on a daily basis and provided extensive help with her care. Throughout the narrative, Jean Denecke explicitly describes the process of solving various functional problems such as turning in bed, lifting a cup to her lips, and hiring and supervising household workers who bore responsibility both for her care and for domestic chores under her supervision. This intimate recitation continues to illustrate for others who survived polio that life can be fulfilling and satisfying with appropriate supports, ingenuity, and creativity. Her story also illustrates how little information and practical assistance was available to help support and guide her reentry until she went to the Georgia Warm Springs Polio Foundation for rehabilitation. Nowhere does she mention seeking or receiving assistance from occupational or physical therapists before her admission there. These disciplines have evolved over the years since she contracted polio and today, their practitioners provide information about assistive devices and strategies for independent living for people with disabilities. Jean Denecke, however, had to discover her own solutions trough trial and error.

Jean Denecke provides a straightforward description of her state of mind as she copes with the details of regaining control over her life and reasserting her authority over her household. Her primary goal of presenting her experience as a guide also limits the extent to which she is willing to reveal or perhaps even explore in any depth the complex, contradictory, and potentially confounding emotions that inevitably accompany such a profound life transition. Rather than detracting from the narrative, however, this tactic enhances our appreciation of the historical period in which her story takes place where social conventions established boundaries that defined what information about family life could comfortably be revealed publicly and what was to remain private. These boundaries are clearly illustrated when she describes in detail how she solves the problem of toileting, but she never tells us, for example, how or if she and her husband found ways to be sexual. Similarly, we are not offered insight into his reaction to the news that his young wife had acquired a significant disability that not only would reshape her life but that surely must have transformed his hopes and expectations for his own future and the future of his family.

For Jean Denecke and many others who contracted polio in the 1940s and 1950s, the opportunity to go to the Georgia Warm Springs Polio Foundation for rehabilitation proved to be life changing. Franklin D. Roosevelt, who had contracted polio and who found that the warm waters of the Georgia resort provided relief from some of the residual effects of polio, founded the hospital at Warm Springs, Georgia in 1927. For the first time since she had contracted polio, at Warm Springs, Jean Denecke was outfitted with an appropriate wheelchair, arm slings, and a custom-made corset, which provided much needed abdominal support that enabled her to sit for longer periods and to breathe more easily. As a patient at Warm Springs, she was the beneficiary of the Foundation's expertise as the leading rehabilitation facility in the country for people with polio. The facility offered a multi-faceted and progressive approach to rehabilitation that fostered the expectation that polio survivors would return to their communities and resume their roles as students, homemakers, workers, and community leaders. While pity was the prevailing community reaction to people with disabilities and disability public policy fostered their segregation from schools and jobs, Warm Springs created a vibrant culture of inclusion and empowerment. Jean Denecke, immersed in this environment during her stay at Warm Springs, not only benefited from medical and rehabilitative interventions, she also bolstered her determination to resume the life she had lived before contracting polio. The Warm Springs culture was infectious. Most former patients went on to lead everyday lives that included marriage, children, and careers. Others, building

on the Warm Springs can-do experience, became key players in
the nation's disability rights movement that spurred sweeping
social and civil rights reforms.

Spanning the five-year period after she contracted polio,
Jean Denecke's memoir affords an intimate and detailed account
of one woman's strategies for accommodating a fundamentally
altered life. For readers who themselves are polio survivors, the
particulars will remind them of the time in their lives when they
faced the same challenges as well as of the shared experiences
that create such a unique bond among this group. For others,
Jean Denecke's account offers a rich glimpse into the polio
experience and illustrates that, indeed, walking isn't everything.

Mary Lou Breslin

About Mary Lou Breslin

Just as Jean Denecke, Mary Lou Breslin also contracted polio,
but in the 1950s. A polio-quadriplegic who uses a motorized
wheelchair, she too was a patient at the then Georgia Warm
Springs Foundation and later attended the University of Illinois
which was accessible to students with mobility disabilities
thanks to a program for veterans with disabilities that had been
established in the late 1940s. She went on to become active
in the disability rights movement, co-founding the Disability
Rights Education and Defense Fund (DREDF), a leading
national disability rights law and policy center, in 1979 where
she presently serves as senior policy advisor.

Ms. Breslin taught graduate courses at the University of
San Francisco, McLaren School of Business, and the University
of California at Berkeley. For eight years, she served as editor
and researcher with the Disability Rights and Independent
Living Project of the Regional Oral History Office of the
Bancroft Library, University of California at Berkeley. She has
written and published on various disability rights topics, most

recently on health care and disability. She received the prestigious Henry B. Betts award in 2002 for improving the lives of people with disabilities. She also received the Paul A. Hearne Award from the Physical and Mental Disability Rights Committee of the American Bar Association in 2000 and a Mary E. Switzer Merit Fellowship in 1995 with the United States Department of Education.

I Get It

To start at the beginning, my daughter Kristin had always been quite healthy until she began to have one throat infection after another. This chronic throat condition led us to have her tonsils removed in 1946 when she was two years old.

When Kris started with a high fever in the middle of September 1947, the first thing I thought of was a sore throat. We took her to our pediatrician immediately and she was started on Sulpha. However, she did not respond to medication, as she usually did. After three days, she was still running a flexible fever, though not high enough for us to become too alarmed.

I had been sleeping with Kris and in the middle of one night, she wakened me with a piercing scream that brought her father on the run from the other bedroom, and she told us that her leg hurt her. We did not turn on the light in her room, and we thought she had had a nightmare. I rubbed her leg and tried to soothe her. She finally calmed down and we all went back to sleep.

When we awakened in the morning and Harry came in, I told him that our bed felt a little strange. I thought that perhaps Kris had wet the bed because of her nightmare. I got up and found that Kris had had diarrhea, and she and I were both a mess. I disrobed the two of us and we got into a tub of hot water while Harry stripped the bed and soaked the linens. Kris had apparently had a muscle spasm during the night that caused the diarrhea. We decided years later that this incident could have had a great deal to do with my getting polio. She did not have any more leg pains or diarrhea, so we forgot about the entire incident.

A few days later, I came up with many aches and pains in my body, and I was particularly conscious of a slight pain in my chest, which made me recall that I had had similar pains a couple of weeks previous. I had thought at the time that I had been smoking too much. I guess I took a couple of aspirin and rested when I could. The next day was a workday for my husband, so I forced myself to get up and get dressed, and as Kris seemed to be better, I dressed her, too.

Later that morning, I decided to call a doctor, since I was not feeling at all as I should. He came out and told me I had pleurisy. Since Kris cried when he started to look at her and her temperature was down that morning, I did not urge him to examine her. The doctor left a prescription for me and advised that I rest as much as possible.

I took my pills faithfully, but I found I was much sicker the next morning. By that time, I had developed excruciating pain in my upper legs and my spine. I went from chills to sweats, and Harry fought a losing battle trying to keep dry pajamas on me. It was a continuous orgy of chills, sweats, oblivion, and horrible racing pains. Through it all, I was concerned for Kris whenever I was awake, and since she was still running a flexible temperature, I asked Harry to make an appointment to take her to our throat specialist.

Harry and my mother took Kris down to the specialist. That was the day I had a stiff neck and could not get my chin down to my chest. At this point, I just knew I had polio. Harry had the doctor check our daughter for polio at my insistence. He came home and said that her reflexes were fine and the doctor's opinion was that she did not have polio.

My mind eased a little bit after that, and I tried to rationalize that perhaps the flu, if that was what I had, might have caused my stiff neck. The things I did not understand, though, were the worsening pains and the fact that it was difficult to breathe when I was not lying on my back. I also noticed that my voice seemed to be very small and weak. I thought at the time that weakness of my body from the fever and pain caused my voice to be weak, but of course, I know now that the respiratory muscles were beginning to be affected.

On Thursday, the day before I went to the hospital, I spent a good part of the day pacing up and down the living room with my new fur coat on trying to take my mind off the horrible pain that I was having. The day had been exhausting. The chills, sweats, and pains were with me constantly until I felt that something, one way or the other, had to happen soon. I did not much care which way, just so I got some relief.

We tried all day to get the doctor, but he was attending a local convention. All we got were promises of a phone call, so we just waited.

I managed to get out to the living room that evening, propped my legs up on a chair, and went to sleep. I had sent Harry to bed, for he was exhausted from caring for his two patients. It turned out that he needed that sleep for the nightmare that was to follow.

When I awakened and started back to the bedroom, delirium had begun to take its effect, so I did not realize that paralysis had set in. I remember that I had quite a struggle stumbling and weaving through the hall, but I finally made it and fell into bed. I can remember feeling glad that I had not tried to waken Harry.

When I awoke the next morning, I felt so much better because all the pains were gone. All of a sudden, however, I realized that I could not move my right leg. I let out a shriek for Harry, and I had him get me up, hang onto me, and I was going to try to walk, but I just could not. Harry sat me down on the bed and, of course, he did not hold me after I sat down. As soon as he let go, I fell right back onto the bed.

We were two scared people, though strangely enough in our anxiety, we just automatically called the doctor, who was in this time, and my mother. We told them both I had polio. The doctor arrived first, confirmed our diagnosis, and reported it to the health authorities. He arranged for me to go to one of the various accredited hospitals that accepted polio in our area.

I remember reading an article about such institutions prior to my illness, and this particular hospital was mentioned as being one of the best equipped for handling polio, though it accepted other contagious diseases as well. It was very crowded when I was admitted, and consequently, acute polio was not a novelty. I soon found out that my woes, both mental and physical, were to become my own particular struggle.

CHAPTER 2

I Am Hospitalized

My very frightened mom came to stay with Kris shortly before the ambulance arrived. I smilingly told her that it could be worse, since only one of my legs was paralyzed. I said this with my tongue in my cheek. During my ride to the hospital, and all that day for that matter, I could feel pins and needles going slowly up first one arm and then the other until I was completely paralyzed.

My ride to the hospital was my first experience with ambulances. The man who sat with me en route encouraged me considerably by telling me of all the people he had taken to the hospital in the previous two weeks who thought they had polio and who had come back the same day. He proved his faith in his own statements by waiting at the hospital until I was diagnosed, but he went back with an empty ambulance.

Harry had to leave me in the basement admitting room, and since it was lunchtime, I had to wait for an examination. I was so scared; I lay on the stretcher stiff as a poker and tried hard to be brave. I would have given anything to have Harry standing beside me holding my hand, but the best I could do was to watch his legs as he walked back and forth outside the windows of my room. I had some silly idea that I could make him hear, and I let out a couple of war whoops, but the walls were thicker than my feeble voice at that point and, of course, he did not hear me.

When I finally was wheeled into the examining room, I got the usual spinal tap. The intern who gave it to me must have been an expert, for I did not feel a thing. After he completed the spinal tap, I heard the intern say, "Plus 100," and I asked what he meant. He said simply, "It means you have polio."

Harry's pajamas were taken off me and put in a sack for him to take home, and I was given my choice of a flannel or a muslin gown. I chose the flannel because I had been freezing for the past week.

After I was dressed in the flannel gown, an attendant asked to take my wedding ring. I balked at this, since I have always been sentimental about taking off my wedding ring. However, after finding out that I had to write my name on a paper relieving the hospital of any responsibility if it were lost, I was about to change my mind. The muscles in my hand and arm were affected by that time, and it was quite a struggle to make even chicken scratches. I did sign my name, though, and kept my wedding ring on.

I guess that was all; I was ready to go to the polio floor. An orderly wheeled me to the corridor where Harry was waiting. We said a hasty good-bye and he was told that I would be there at least three weeks. Visiting hours were Wednesday and Sunday. That was Friday and already I was looking forward to Sunday.

I was put in a room with two girls who were still in isolation. One girl was thirteen years old and had been in the hospital just a few days. The other was a young married woman and I believe she had been there two weeks at the time I was admitted.

I still had a sinking feeling in the pit of my stomach, and I watched apprehensively each treatment the other girls were given. When you are in isolation, your therapy is given to you in your room. I watched the therapist give Peggy her treatment first with interest, and then with foreboding, as I heard a couple of exclamations of pain come from Peggy.

There seemed to be someone constantly crying out, and in my anxiety over Kristin every time a child cried, I was sure that Kris had been brought to the hospital and I was not being told. That feeling persisted for several days, but I was finally reassured that she was coming along fine with my mother and dad at their home.

When I was put to bed, I was still able to turn myself over, raise both arms above my head, move one leg, etc. I do not know exactly how long it took me to become completely paralyzed, for there was not a clock in sight. I do know that the gradual loss of strength, and then finally the inability to move at all, was the most terrifying experience I have ever had.

I do not remember supper, but I do remember having chocolate milk some time in the afternoon. I promptly lost the milk in the midst of giving the story of my onset of polio to some young medical student. I had enough paralysis at the time that I had a good deal of difficulty in holding the emesis basin where I needed it, and I was horrified that the medical student had to stand and watch me. I was also disgusted that he did not make any effort to help me. One always reads that nausea is a common accompaniment to polio, but this was the one and only time I ever remember being nauseated. Perhaps this was because I had not eaten, nor did I eat very much in the days to come.

I was trying very hard not to cry, and the few words of conversation I had with the other girls were all speculation on when we could go home. I do not think any of us realized the length of time that it takes to repair damage done by polio. I know it just never occurred to me, even after I was totally paralyzed, that the paralysis would not go away in the same manner in which it had enveloped me.

My own first experience with therapy was late in the evening. The head therapist had come dashing in that afternoon. She said she really should examine me herself but that she did not have time, and I could tell her where I had paralysis.

After supper, I heard a rumbling noise coming down the hall. Whatever was making the noise stopped at our room, and two women came in beside my bed and told me that I was going to get packed. I had already heard from the other two girls in the room that the packs par-boiled you, and I had an idea that the packs were going to miraculously cure me.

Between the time the therapist had asked me where I was paralyzed and the time the packers came in, I had developed more paralysis. When they started to pack me, I was quite insistent that they get more packs for the additional paralysis. I did not realize that each patient as he comes in is given his own individual pack and that each piece of material is cut to fit an individual affected area.

The pack for each affected area consisted of three different layers. The first layer was a piece of fine soft wool; the second was oilskin; and the third layer was a thick, heavy, coarse padding to keep in the heat. If an entire leg was involved, the lower leg was wrapped in one pack and the upper leg in another completely separate pack. The pieces were put on systematically and taken off systematically, so that the packers were able to follow their routine quickly and the packs were not allowed to cool. Only the inner layers of the packs were wrapped together and put into a steamer. Then they were transferred to a washing machine that was wheeled down to the room. The wool pieces were put through the wringer by one worker and handed to one of two women standing on either side of the bed. Then the dry oilskin was put on, followed by the dry heavy covering.

2 - I Am Hospitalized

The packs were extremely hot, but I did not complain because, as I said before, I thought the packs were going to cure me. I figured that the hotter they were, the more quickly they could do their work. After I got out of the packs, I noticed that I seemed to be having a lot of trouble breathing, and I was not talking very loud. I did not want to frighten the thirteen-year-old girl in the next bed, but I finally asked her if it was hot in the room and if she had any trouble getting her breath. The feeling I had was similar to that one gets on a very humid day—a breathless feeling is the best description I can offer for the sensation.

When my little friend gave me a negative answer to my question, I asked her if she could hear me plainly—that I seemed to be having trouble making my voice come out. When I got my second "no," I told her I thought there was something wrong and asked her if she would please call a nurse.

There was not a signal system on that floor, so when one wanted something, one opened one's mouth and shouted. One of the attendants came in and I told her my trouble. I was panicky by that time, and when no one else came in a few minutes, I had my little friend call again for me. She startled me when, after calling for a nurse, she said to me, "You're probably going to be put into a respirator." She had picked up the hospital vernacular readily and her term "respirator" did not mean iron lung to me, as it should have. I asked her in a puzzled way if I would be coming back to that room in the morning. She said, "Oh no! Once you're put in a respirator, you're in one for a long time."

Walking Isn't Everything

CHAPTER 3

I Am Put in
an Iron Lung

When the attendant came back the second time, she had a nurse with her, and they wheeled my bed out into the hall alongside an iron lung. As much as I had read about it, the significance of the iron lung did not occur to me at the time. The resident physician had been called to the floor and after a conference with the nurse, he helped an orderly lift me into the iron lung. After the machine was operating, the doctor told me that they were putting me in the iron lung so that I could get a good night's sleep. Strangely enough, I seemed to relax after I was put in the respirator, and I started to doze off.

Harry had gone home after I was taken up to the polio floor, and he found my mother and father and a friend of theirs who was a nurse busily disinfecting our house and furnishings. They had my bed out in the yard scrubbing it with Lysol; everything that could be boiled was boiled and other things discarded. In the midst of their efforts, they had a visit from a representative of the Wayne County Health Department who was surprised at the efficiency of the work being done, until she learned that both my mother and her friend were nurses themselves.

My folks went home that evening, and Harry said it was almost midnight when a call came from the hospital telling him that he should come immediately. He had to call my folks to come back to the house to stay with Kris. Harry was pacing up and down in front of the house when my folks arrived, and my mother wanted my father to go with Harry. However, she was shaking so badly that my father refused to leave her, so Harry dashed off alone. As soon as he was gone, my mother called Harry's father, because they were all sure that either I was dead or about to die, and Mother did not think Harry should go through that alone.

When I was put in the iron lung, I was told matter-of-factly that they knew I would want to see my husband, so they had sent for him. As sick as I was, I finally realized how close to death I must be, or they would not have sent for Harry. While I had no exact idea what time it was, I was sure it must be late at night.

Harry and his father both came, put on gowns, and stood outside my open door. I guess I did most of the talking. I kept telling them I was not going to die but as soon as they left, I am afraid that I was not quite so brave. The night nurse brought me several cups of hot tea, trying to quiet my shakes and tears. That was the beginning of many nights of not being able to get my mind to light on any particular thing. I seemed to realize then that things could never be as they had been in the past, and I surely did not know what the future would bring.

CHAPTER 4

Polio Woes

E ven though I was still on the critical list the next day, I received packs. However, this time, it was much more of an ordeal than it had been the night before. I could no longer breathe outside the iron lung, nor did I have enough breath to operate my vocal chords. The packers had quite a time quickly pulling the respirator apart, putting one pack on, and then slamming the respirator together again to give me a breath, until eventually, they had put on a complete pack.

When I was packed that afternoon, I felt concentrated heat on my left arm and left hip. When I asked, not meaning to be argumentative, "You wouldn't burn me, would you?" the packers assured me that they would not. However, when the pack was removed, my lower arm was quite badly burned, and so was my hip. From the looks of the scars, the pack must have been put on wrinkled.

Plain Vaseline was applied to my burns. Therapy on that arm was limited and packs were discontinued for several weeks. I apparently lay un-noticed with my arm upon my chest and my ring finger and my little finger bent under for the time that it took for the burns to heal. The result was a crooked arm and bent fingers, which I still have. It is my opinion that if hand splints had been used early, the deformity would not have occurred.

The critical list still had my name on it the next week, and that week, my iron lung broke down in the middle of the night. The nurse had opened the respirator for the bedpan, and when she closed the respirator again, it did not turn on. Orderlies are used to such emergencies even if patients are not. A good, strong, husky one was immediately found to hand-pump the respirator until another one could be moved up to the floor and made up. It had all happened very quickly, and it was handled so efficiently that I did not have time to get scared until it was all over and I had been moved to the other respirator. I was quite upset after the transfer and could not get to sleep. My burns had gotten the worst of it in the move, and they hurt badly.

I think this might be a good place to explain that polios have very acute feeling, because the disease does not affect the sensory nerves. In early polio, the muscles are extremely sore, and in my case, the involvement was so extensive that my body was like one continuous bruise to touch. It is not hard to imagine the pain involved in having three people slide me out of one iron lung, carry me, and slide me into another. Every nerve I had left must have been on edge, for I really was in a dilemma the rest of the night. It might not have been so bad if I had been able to move around as one often does on a restless night. But all I could do was lie there; when it got too bad, cry; and then call for someone to move a leg or arm or a foot.

After I was moved to the new respirator, I felt sure that I had a chain around my neck, and I kept trying to tell nurses and attendants just where the chain hurt me. Whether or not this was delirium, I do not know. Nevertheless, the next day, one of the supervisors hit upon the idea that perhaps the mattress was not long enough in the respirator to which I had been moved, for I am quite tall. After the night I had just gone through, I was willing to try anything, so I went through the discomfort of being moved into yet another iron lung to which the original mattress had been transferred. The mattress change helped a lot, and though it was weeks before I got a good night's sleep, I did not have another night quite as bad as that one.

The day the doctors first saw my intercostal muscles move, exactly nine days after I was admitted, was really a joyous day for me. I was told it probably meant that eventually I would be able to get out of the iron lung. This realization came to me with a bit of shock as well as joy, for I am sure I had been much too ill up to this point to realize that if those intercostal muscles did not return, I would have to spend the rest of my life in an iron lung. This has happened in a number of cases. However, the return of these muscles was real, and every one on the floor had to be told. I could hardly wait for Harry to come that evening so I could tell him, for it was a day of real hope for me.

I thought I was on the road to full recovery for sure, and I was so enthusiastic even the next week, that I made myself very unpopular. The fifteen-year-old girl in the next room was being taken out of her respirator and laid on the bed for increasingly longer periods. One day, I commented that she should be able to go home in another month.

I realize now that my knowledge of polio at that time was very limited, but no new patient is willing or capable of thinking of long hospitalization. My comments about going home were apparently overhead and passed on. The next afternoon, the head therapist visited me and informed me that if I thought June would be going home in another month, I was mistaken. I was told that she would do well if she was home in six months, and as for myself, I would be doing extremely well if I made it home in a year.

I kept my face straight until Harry came, but our visiting hour that evening was full of tears. I was all for going home right then and there. I think I made up my mind then that I was not going to stay in that hospital for a year.

This incident, as far as I am concerned, was much too big a thought, given to me too early and too abruptly, and resulted in nothing but rebellion. It was an unfortunate incident, and the ensuing mental attitude with which it left me was as much a handicap as my physical condition for a long time to come. I have since tried to analyze the incident. I have concluded that no doubt, I had done a good job of keeping my emotions under control to the casual observer, and the therapist was far too busy to notice the undercurrent of emotions that were dammed up inside me. Her statement just caused a flood of confused emotions, and I had been too recently close to death to be ready to accept the thought of a year's hospitalization without rebellion.

Perhaps again, if my involvement had not been so extensive, the jolt into reality would not have packed such a wallop. Then I would have had some morsel of independence on which to fall back. As it was, though, I was completely dependent upon others. I had even lost my formal name, for from the time I was wheeled onto the polio floor, I was addressed as Jean, never as Miss Denecke. The quick familiarity bothered me, especially since most of the attendants themselves were known as Miss or Miss

CHAPTER 5

I Am Learning

It took me some time to become aware of the structure of my respirator apart from the audible whoosh sound that the bellows made as it continuously pumped air in and out. I learned that when the reading on a pressure gauge on top of the machine would drop below the number at which it usually operated, I would feel that I was not getting as deep a breath as usual. I also learned that an emergency bell attached to this pressure gauge would give a warning ring if the pressure should accidently be cut off or reach a dangerous low.

There had to be a way to adjust the patient without pulling the iron lung apart each time, so the designer had made two little doors on each side of the respirator which, when opened, showed a sponge rubber disk about one-half inch thick with a hole in the middle of it. This enabled an attendant to put his hand through the opening. The attendant's wrist and arm would seal the opening, and there was not a great reduction of pressure. These doors were called portholes.

A much larger third door, when open, did not have the rubber disk. Consequently, the pressure was greatly reduced when it was necessary to use that opening for a larger workable area. However, the pressure was not reduced to the degree it would have been had the whole machine been opened. This door also was made of glass to enable one to see into the respirator.

The inside of the respirator was fitted with a most comfortable foam rubber mattress, and since all polio patients must use a footboard so that they do not get the well-known drop foot, mine was so equipped.

The opening for the head followed the same principle as the doors, for there was a large rubber disk, or collar, with a small opening for the head to go through. This opening could be enlarged, for there were three leather straps which, when put through the rubber collar opening and pulled tight, held the collar open to head size. After the head was through the opening, the leather straps were released so that the collar fit closely around the neck, thereby sealing that opening for the same reason that I have explained above.

Every iron lung was fitted with a mirror to enable the patient to see what was going on behind him. Those of us in respirators had many chuckles over the fact that every visiting day always brought curious visitors to the door with comments about having to lie and watch one's self all day long. Fortunately, it was impossible for the patient to see himself in this mirror.

About this time, I became acquainted with physical therapy in earnest. Of course, everyone knows that physical therapy plays a very important part in the muscle rehabilitation of every person who has had polio. It is amazing how tight one's muscles can become in just a few days.

My physical therapist had worked at Percy Jones Hospital in Battle Creek, Michigan, and she was well qualified in every sense of the word. She explained to me as she went along that to begin with, she would have to work through the portholes in my respirator until my respiratory muscles became strong enough for me to be out of the iron lung for at least short periods. She had a set of routine exercises that she went through, and if a certain portion of my body was tight, that portion was moved and held to this point of tightness and pushed a little harder each day until the point of flexibility that she desired was achieved.

Each muscle that had been affected had to be re-educated, which required intense concentration and cooperation on the part of the patient. My therapist was a very understanding and helpful person. She surely realized that each time she gave me that little extra push she was giving me a good-sized pain at the same time, and one that sometimes was remembered until the next day.

When you first become a polio victim, you are so anxious to get well that I think any adult would gladly take anything in the line of treatment to get well. I know that was my whole attitude in spite of being so very sick and probably not always coherent. A day did not pass that I did not ask my therapist if she thought I was taking enough pain and if I was cooperating to the utmost. In those early days, there was no sign of improvement, except perhaps in my respiratory muscles. I still could not move but one arm, the right one, and when I lifted that, I could not get it back down without walking it down. This was accomplished by wriggling the wrist and using the fingers at the same time.

In my first days of therapy, the treatment lasted probably a half-hour. The days began to assume a pattern with breakfast over and packs ready to begin at 8:00 A.M. I was packed all morning right up until lunchtime, and then there was a rest hour between 1:00 and 2:00 P.M. Packs started again at 2:00 P.M. and went on until about 4:30 P.M. Since my therapy treatment was given frequently during the rest hour, I did not miss the routine series of packs that were given during the afternoon.

After the supper hour, patients in respirators were allowed visitors from 6:00 to 6:30 P.M. every day. This one thing carried me through that horrible six months. If I was not packed in the evening, and not many patients were, I just lay there and looked at the ceiling until it was time for someone to come in and fix me up for the night.

The hospital had only three projected books, and since I did not get polio until October, all of the projectors were being used. I spent so many of my evenings crying that one intern took pity on me and borrowed a projected book from a kind patient. Since I was not able to push the button that turned the pages at the time, the intern fixed it so I could turn the pages by pushing the button with my chin. I have always loved to read, and that pastime was a welcome diversion. I read the complete library of the hospital's projected books, including Bates' edition of the Bible.

There were many nights in the hospital when it just seemed that sleep never would come. When you cannot move yourself and your body has polio soreness, each little wrinkle feels like a mountain under you. One of my friends who is a nurse compared me to the story of "The Princess and the Pea."

It seemed like there was always some adjustment needed. Although I did not mean to be asking for constant attention, what always seemed like at least an hour since I had needed something, in reality was closer to fifteen minutes. By the time I would think that I was comfortable and was ready to settle down and go to sleep, thoughts would start racing through my mind, and the first thing I knew, there were tears racing down my cheeks. My nose would suddenly need blowing, the pillow would be soggy, and of course, it was impossible to repair the damage that the tears had done. The truth of the matter is, in looking back over it, that it was just a case of being downright scared to death. I think in the first four weeks that I was a polio patient, I did not average four hours sleep a night, and that alone would indicate what a pain in the neck I must have been.

Throughout this four-week period of night restlessness, one of the nurses, who was a staff instructor and who came in to see me most every day, had been urging for me to have a special nurse. Finally, one of the day attendants was assigned to sit with me at night.

Miss Daly was a colored woman and one of the kindest persons I have ever known. The first night she sat with me, I wanted her to talk to me and stay in the room with me constantly. I think I could have talked to her all night long if she had not finally insisted that I try to get some sleep. It was like having a private nurse. She did things for me cheerfully, and I did not have the feeling that I was taking her attention from some other patient when I asked her for something.

During the period when I was having such a frightfully difficult time at night, Harry had offered to get a private nurse for me but for some reason or other, the hospital had discouraged it. About three days after Miss Daly came on night duty, I settled down and started to sleep. It was about that time that we got another respirator patient in, a woman about my age, and Miss Daly was assigned to take care of her also. As I listened to the new patient's constant calling, I was well enough to relive those early agonies of sleeplessness and want. She was indeed fortunate to have had Miss Daly available to her in her early sickness.

During almost every polio season, one reads that an expectant mother has become a victim of polio. While I was in the hospital, a woman was brought in who was well along in her eight month of pregnancy. Everyone on the floor was concerned for her and the baby, and those of us who could see her room watched with eagle eyes for any unusual activity. One morning about a week after she arrived, I saw her being wheeled out on a stretcher, and it was not long before news came from the delivery room that she had had a healthy baby boy. The baby stayed in the maternity ward and the mother returned to the polio floor.

As the days passed, my therapy treatments were increased, for I was able to breathe without the aid of the respirator for longer periods. That meant that my respirator could be opened and left open while the treatment was given.

Then came the day when I was taken out of the iron lung, put on a stretcher, and wheeled down to the therapy room to be put on a table. It was probably only a matter of being wheeled three doors down the hall, but it was quite a frightening experience to be out of sight of the iron lung and wondering if your next breath was going to come all right.

One would think I had been wheeled a mile on that stretcher from all the thoughts that went through my mind, but I can also remember getting glimpses of strange faces and wondering what new "stretch" was going to come my way since all of me would be exposed.

The cart was pulled up alongside a therapy table, and I was rolled from the cart to the table. When you cannot help yourself, you have a constant fear of falling that is beyond explanation, except to say that it was the most real fear that I have ever experienced.

I just knew I was going to keep right on rolling and fall off that table, although it had taken quite a mighty heave to get me off the stretcher in the first place. The table was a far cry from lying on my sponge rubber respirator mattress, and I knew then for sure that I had lost a lot of padding. I lived through the therapy treatment, but I am sure that I was not concentrating on muscle coordination much that day.

After the first trip to the therapy room, my time out of the iron lung became an established matter. Each Saturday, the hospital medical director would make the rounds and check the chart on the wall, which recorded my pulse rate before and after I was taken from the respirator. The time started with fifteen minutes out and generally increased fifteen minutes a week.

I was put into the iron lung on October 3, 1947, and I said goodbye to it permanently on June 1, 1948. There was no time that I remember that I every backslid as far as time out of the respirator was concerned.

After I had been in the hospital for three or four weeks, I was visited one day by the head therapist and an intern who brought in a machine known as a spirometer. This is a device by which a patient's vital capacity is measured. The intern explained that the rubber mouthpiece that was attached to a long hose would be put in my mouth and I was to take a good deep breath and blow as hard as I could. The vital capacity would be recorded on the graph that was also attached to the machine. Vital capacity means the amount of air the patient is capable of drawing into his lungs.

After two or three blows, I was told that the graph registered a mere 200. I was full of questions, and I found out that a normal person blew anywhere from 1500 on up. Since I had been in the iron lung a few weeks, I had been thinking that I was improving rapidly as far as my respiratory muscles were concerned. I could not help but ask what they thought my vital capacity would have registered when I went into the iron lung. The intern told me he would estimate it at 50.

In a way, that was a black day for me, for in figure comparison, I did not show up very well. Those vital capacity tests were given periodically. They measured when you were first taken from the iron lung and the rapidity with which you were able to leave the machine. The last time I had a vital capacity test, I blew 850, but I have been assured that it is much higher now.

Walking Isn't Everything

CHAPTER 6

Highs and Lows

Kristen had her fourth birthday before Christmas, and Harry brought me three snapshots of my cocker spaniel and her, which I had taped to my mirror. It seemed longer than ten weeks since I had seen her, and I was so lonesome that day and very rebellious about the whole situation.

Then came Christmas, and that was another disappointment. It was a bitter blow when they told us that visiting hours would be from 9:00 to 10:30 A.M. on Christmas Day. Of course, my folks wanted to see me then and so did Harry, and it meant they would all have to arise at an extremely early hour so that Kris could have her Christmas celebration first. Four-year-olds just are not old enough to wait to open presents, for any reason.

All the patients on our floor had gone home except the four girls in the iron lungs, and none of us could understand why visiting hours had to be at such an unreasonable hour. We kept hoping until the last minute that someone would have a change of heart.

Just before visiting hours, a nurse came through with some beautiful dolls that the Goodfellows had dressed. There had been a few left after distribution to the children in the hospital, so she offered a doll to each of us four "respirator" girls. I chose a little blonde-haired doll dressed in a beautiful yellow poplin dress for Harry to take home to Kris.

My folks came in to see me first, and when their half-hour of the visiting period was up, they went down to the car where Harry was waiting with Kris. They went on home while Harry visited with me. I was not happy at all, and I am afraid I did not do much to make Christmas very happy for my family. I was feeling sorry for myself about that time.

New Year's Eve was like any other night with bedtime at the usual early hour. By January, some of the better patients were allowed up and used to come, stand by the door, and talk with those of us who could not get up. Misery loves company, and we all had many miseries to share.

I guess I was not the only polio patient who had been depressed by the holidays. In January, the girls who were mothers were told that they could see their children in the basement of the hospital for an hour every other Saturday. Naturally, I said yes, I wanted to see Kris, but the closer the time came, the more qualms I had about the advisability of it.

I had seen myself in the mirror a few times, and something horrible had happened to my complexion. I do not think you could put a finger between blackheads and blemishes on my face, neck, and shoulders and I had lost a tremendous amount of weight. My hair was not hiding the shampoos it had been given with green soap, either, and my hairstyle was far from flattering since it was combed straight back. Besides my difficulty in speaking and obvious paralysis, I knew that I would not be the Mommy that Kris remembered.

However, my curiosity about my daughter won the argument I was having with myself. On the Saturday designated for her visit, I had asked one of the student nurses well in advance to powder, comb me, and fix me up. My folks had brought me a gardenia that morning, and I felt that I smelled pretty even if I did not look very pretty.

My worries were all in vain. Kris came tearing in the door, said hello, looked the stretcher over, and then noticed the open door into the next room where she heard one of the other patient's little boys galloping around. It did not take her long to get over to the door and ask the little boy to come out. They spent most of the next hour racing back and forth and even made it back to the kitchen and came out with cookies. Wheeling the stretcher serves as a pastime, too, and I was glad that it was not my first time on a stretcher when she started pushing me around. She looked fine and I managed to keep back the tears during her visit. Kris visited me three times while I was in the hospital.

I would like to explain my wonderful and satisfactory relationship with the National Foundation for Infantile Paralysis and our county chapter of that organization. Shortly after I was admitted to the hospital and the financial arrangements were being made, Harry was told about the workings of the foundation and made an appointment with the case coordinator for our city.

Harry told her that we were buying our home and that he had been in the army for almost five years. Anyone who knows army life knows that there is not a great deal of money to be saved during time spent in the service. Harry was assured that I would receive proper care and that they did not want us to have to sell our house, thereby making it necessary to lower our standard of living to a great degree. He had hospitalization insurance and we used that to the limits of the policy.

This early reassurance and help was a tremendous load off my husband's mind. At the time that I first became ill, there were so many big things to cope with that it was a real relief not to have the financial burden, too. From that day to this, we have always had the helping hand of the Foundation to help us meet the needs of each new phase of life with polio. We have tried to do our best too, so that I would not become too big a burden for the Foundation.

About this time, I began to have my first real wrestles with physical therapy. I think my shoulders gave me the most trouble, because they had become quite tight through inability to exercise to a great degree because of the iron lung. The aim of the therapist was to get my arms to lie back flat on the table over my head.

I was apparently unusually tight and had an extremely low threshold of pain. The combination of these two at the time just seemed insurmountable because the pain was so intense. In one of my treatments, I was stretched to the point where the side of my breast was black and blue. For days after that, I could have let out a scream if my arm was touched, had I had the strength to do so.

I noticed that many patients had the ability to open their mouths and scream, where I did not. I would cry and tighten up inside, so that I could not relax, which made it all the worse. It seemed like all of my waking hours were spent dreading the next treatment. They tried Phenobarbital with me, but it did not seem to help very much.

In spite of the therapist's efforts and mine too, the medical director, when he saw me out on the bed one Saturday, told me that I was not stretching out fast enough and that I would have to take more pain and more stretching. I began to cry and protest that I was taking about as much stretching as I could. The doctor gave me a pep talk, but I was so terrified that I was beyond reasoning. I could not think of anything else

56

but the pain that faced me. I had had so much already that I felt I was at the breaking point mentally. My recovery had been so slow, except for the improvement in my respiratory muscles, that I felt everything was just hopeless.

Every polio patient goes through a phase of not wanting to live, and I was no exception, to say the very least. Looking back on it now, I know that this phase was much more difficult for Harry really, than it was for me. Up to the point when I decided in earnest that I wanted to die, Harry had worked out a routine that he seemed to believe in—that approximately every third to fifth day, my spirits would be at an extremely low ebb.

As the days wore on, though, it seemed that every visiting hour brought bitter, bitter words to my mouth. My particular plan to die involved having Harry bring some rat poisoning to me at the hospital. I do not quite know why it had to be rat poisoning, for we had never had any rats or poisoning around our house. At some time or other, I must have read too many whodunits. However, that was my decision and that was what I wanted Harry to bring. I told him that I did not want to see him if he did not bring the poison; I said I never wanted to see our daughter again, and that to me life was just a hopeless mess. I do not ever remember being resentful or envious of other people's good health; I just wanted to die and get away from it all.

All the good things that have ever been said about the very best of people could certainly be said of my husband, for he weathered that very difficult period with me. Very frequently, he gave me the good argument for which I apparently was looking. He did not try to mollycoddle me in any way or to offer false hope. Sometimes, I do not understand how he was able to come every visiting hour as he did and listen to what he must have taken from me. However, we both learned in time that with polio, things have a way of working out for everyone, if they can just pull together and have patience with one another until fate's plan begins to take shape.

Walking Isn't Everything

CHAPTER 7

The Beginnings of Determination

Entertainment was always welcome at the hospital, and it was something that was rarely offered. One of my friends approached The Four Dukes, a local comedy-singing quartet, about the possibility of putting on a performance one Sunday afternoon for the polio patients. I had seen them several times before I became ill, and when the quartet agreed to do a show, there was quite a lot of anticipation among the patients.

This was in January, the month of the March of Dimes fund-raising drive for the National Foundation for Infantile Paralysis. On the day of the performance, a photographer from one of the local papers came in and took some pictures of The Four Dukes and two of the patients in respirators.

The show gave everyone a big boost. One of our youngest patients was a blond, blue-eyed, angelic-looking boy under two years of age. When the boys sang "Kentucky Babe" to that little lad in his crib, one of the performers had tears running down his cheeks as he thought of his own boy of approximately the same age.

We also had a few movies that were brought in by the father of one of the patients. When we "went" to the movies, it was a lot of work for the attendants, since movies were shown in the hall. Wheelchairs had to be rounded up for those who could sit in them long enough to watch a movie, stretchers for those who could not. If the respirator patients had their time out for the day, the machine and patients were shoved into the hall and extension cords added.

It was quite a problem to arrange those respirators so they were not in the viewing line of the other patients. There was always at least one iron lung at each movie. The movies were never long, because each patient had to be made ready for bed before the afternoon and early evening crew went off duty.

Another new experience was that of sitting up in a wheelchair for the first time. The chair that I was to be put in was one of those old-fashioned wooden cane-backed chairs, and I found myself fighting with mixed emotions about whether or not I was anxious to get into a wheelchair. By that time, I was quite confident of my ability to breathe out of the iron lung, but I must say that when I got into the chair, I really knew I was breathing on my own.

In my own mind, I seriously doubted that the attendants could ever get me into that wheelchair, but they assured me that they had put more than one polio patient into one. After the chair was well padded with pillows, I closed my eyes tightly and kept them closed until I heard someone say "There." I opened my eyes and found myself in an upright position.

It took a few minutes to be settled so that I was able to talk, and I learned that it is a lot easier to breathe when you are lying down than it is when you are sitting up. Every breath that I took was a tremendous effort and I was aware that each breath was an extremely shallow one.

I was able to see part of my feet and my toes, and they were a sorry looking sight. They looked very puffy and were all colors, with blue and black predominating. I noticed that my fingers were crooked, and I thought to myself that if my hands ever stopped shaking long enough for me to hold a cup again, my little finger on my right hand would have the accepted crook to it.

I noticed the scar from the burn on my left lower arm, and that, too, was many colors and not very nice to look at. I do not think that I was up long enough that day to ask for a mirror to see what the rest of me looked like, for my sitting up amounted to only a very few minutes and I was more than glad to get in a prone position again.

The first time I was put up in a wheelchair for visiting hours was quite an occasion, and that time I had to have a mirror and some make-up put on. Breathing still was not any easier for me when I was sitting up, even though I had been up several times before I was allowed to try to sit up for a short part of the visiting hour.

I remember that I did not have breath enough to give Harry my usual sales talk on bringing the rat poison.

Sitting up gave me quite a few conflicting emotions with which to wrestle. It was something I wanted to do very badly, but when I got up, I was so uncomfortable that I wanted to get back to bed as quickly as possible. The effort I had to make to breathe and sit up was tremendously weakening. During that time, I felt so good lying down and so bad when I got up that I could not see any improvement at all. It would be difficult to set down all the thoughts that came to my mind. I was not able to be out of the respirator for about five or six hours, and I began to feel that perhaps I could get well faster if I were at home.

Walking Isn't Everything

CHAPTER 8

Home Again

I began to wonder how things could be worked out if I were able to convince everyone that I should go home. I believe it was about this time that I began talking more about going home and less about rat poison. When I look back now over the tremendous undertaking it was to make the move, I wonder on which topic Harry preferred to hear me dissertate. He certainly must have admitted to himself the severity of my polio and he must have known that I was not going to make any spectacular recovery in any short time.

I still had my fears of therapy, and I am afraid that I presented quite a problem to my own therapist. News had gotten around, via the grapevine, about how one of the head therapists would occasionally come in to check a patient, and during her examination, she would stretch the patient to the point where he or she would not forget it for a while. That is what started to happen to me one morning before breakfast.

I had not finished my breakfast when the packers came in to start the day's packs, and I asked to be excused for the bedpan before they got started. Just after I was put on the bedpan, the therapist I had been hearing about came into my room and started manipulating one of my arms. I told her that I was slightly indisposed and asked if she would please postpone her examination for a few minutes. She apparently preferred to continue, and after some flippant remark, continued to do just that.

When I asked her again, a little more emphatically this time, if she would please wait, she threw my arm on the bed and said, "I don't care if you ever get well!" Everyone in the room was speechless, and of course, I burst into tears. I guess she had so adequately voiced what I had been thinking myself that the whole episode upset me very much.

I was excused from treatment that day, and by the time Harry came that evening, I had worked myself into quite a state. Harry had been having trouble enough trying to convince me that I was better off in the hospital than I would have been at home, and this new situation did not help him any.

Harry went over to see the medical director who was in charge of the hospital. The doctor and Harry agreed that my encounter with the head therapist had been indeed an untimely happening, and that perhaps it would be better if I did go home. My time out of the respirator had been increasing as per the schedule that had been planned for me, but the doctor suggested that I stay until I was able to be out of the lung entirely, which would have been six to eight more weeks. I was extremely anxious to get home, though, and I had thought about it so much that I just knew it would work out. I finally succeeded in convincing Harry to let me try it.

We began to make plans for me to go home, but I tried not to say anything to anyone around the hospital. Perhaps this was because I did not want anyone to try to discourage me. The word did leak out, though, and there were varied comments around the hospital.

One does not make many friends with other patients after having a bad attack of polio because it is impossible to get around. For that reason, I did not have any fond farewells to make when I left the hospital. One of the attendants who had been planning to leave the hospital anyway had agreed to take care of me at home for a while. The working arrangements that I made with her were more agreeable to her home life at the time than what she had at the hospital. She was very familiar with my iron lung and my routine hot packs, and she was confident that she could care for me.

During these months of emotional upset, I developed a very aggressive bowel condition. I had practically no control at all, but the fact that it was not prevalent when I first got polio led us to feel that in time it would clear up. By the time I was ready to go home, this condition had cleared up almost completely. When the morning came for me to go home, however, I am afraid the excitement was a little too much for me and once again, I had my old troubles. The condition existed even after I was home for a few months, which made me very unhappy. I think the loss of control of one's bowels is one of the most humiliating situations with which an adult might have to cope.

The Foundation had agreed to loan us the iron lung in our home for as long as I needed it. I had been moved to another iron lung the day before I was to go home so that the one that I was used to would be the one that went to my home. It was washed and rolled to the end of the hall until a truck came for it. It did not leave until about an hour before I was scheduled to leave, and I do not know how many times I asked someone to peek down the hall to see if my iron lung had left yet. I was extremely anxious to go home that morning, but I will readily admit that there were many clouds of doubt hanging over my horizon. However, I guess a strong will to lick them existed in my mind.

We called the same ambulance that took me to the hospital, and strangely enough, the driver and attendant remembered having delivered me to the hospital some six months before. Since Harry had stayed at home to be sure that everything was ready there, my mother rode in the ambulance with me.

It was a nice bright sunny day, and the air was as wonderful as I had thought it would be. I could not see very much on the ride home because I could not roll over or lift my head. Apparently, the neighborhood had been alerted for when we turned down our street, several people were standing on their front porches. When we got down to our corner, a gathering of children was in front of the house.

I could see the truck out in front, loaded with men, which had delivered the respirator. There was also a police cruiser, and I guess it made quite an exciting morning for our neighborhood. When I got up to the porch, I could see Kris bouncing up and down, and I glimpsed my cocker spaniel running around trying to look into the stretcher to see if that was Mama's voice she heard.

Harry had taken up the carpets in the living room, and the iron lung made it through the door and was set up in the living room. I had stood the trip very well and did not need any help from the respirator, so I was carried back to the bedroom where I saw my new bedroom furniture Harry had bought at Christmastime.

Everything was confusion after the ambulance drivers left. Kris and the dog both piled up on the bed, bouncing my legs every which way. I was all wadded up in a robe and the clothing that we had put on so I would not catch cold coming home. My toes were smashed down by the covers, but through it all, I was not saying a word about anything. I was just happy to be home.

We finally decided that I had better be straightened out, and Harry was pleased to see that the footboard that he had made for the bed filled the bill. I was made comfortable and settled until it was time for my hours to be spent in the respirator. Some friends came to visit that afternoon, and I received some lovely flowers.

It was a wonderful day, but when it was all over, we agreed that it had been an exhausting one, too. I slept very well that first night at home, and Harry heard me the first time I called when I awoke in the morning.

Walking Isn't Everything

Walking Isn't Everything

CHAPTER 9

A Fresh Start

The Foundation, in addition to loaning me my respirator at home, also sent an electric steamer to be used in preparing my packs, so the next day, we set about establishing a routine that would be convenient to our home life.

My husband worked during the day, but my father and one of our neighbors were working the night shift and they were able to take turns helping to carry me from the respirator to bed each morning. My time out of the respirator had gradually increased to ten hours a day. I would get out of it at approximately 10:00 A.M. and would stay out until 8:00 P.M. It was very easy for two people, even though one was a woman, to get me out of the respirator and into bed. I weighed well under 100 pounds, and my body was not bent when I was carried but was rolled right up to the persons carrying me so that I was almost on my side. The difficulty always came in going around corners and watching that my feet were not bumped.

I started sitting up in a lounge chair, about three times a week as I remember it, trying to increase my sitting up time. I still had to have pillows, even in a lounge chair. I remember telling my mother one time while I was sitting up that if I could only get to the point where I could breathe freely while in a sitting position that I would not ask for another thing.

After I had sat up as long as I felt I should, I would go back to bed, and the woman who was taking care of me would use one or two hot packs on me. We used packs for approximately a month after I came home from the hospital and then we discontinued them.

I had a lot of trouble with my tailbone when I was lying in bed. As I have said before, my respirator was equipped with a sponge rubber mattress. The hospital beds had very thin cotton-filled mattresses, and my tailbone had always bothered me a lot when I was lying in bed at the hospital. But there I had been moved more frequently back and forth to the treatment room, to the bathtub and such, and I did not seem to notice the discomfort to the degree that I did when I got home.

We had a new mattress and springs on our bed, and I had not been home more than a month when one of the springs started to poke up through the ticking because of the constant use. Then we traded mattresses with the other bed, which had a cotton-padded mattress. This was more comfortable than the mattress with springs, but I was still having trouble with pressure points.

One of my neighbors made me some small baby-sized pillows to use under each hip to get the weight off my tailbone and two small elbow pillows to use about an inch off each elbow bone. That too was a severe point of irritation. My arms used to go to sleep, and eventually they would start to burn and pain.

Finally, we invested in a foam rubber mattress and complementary box springs, and we certainly feel that the money was well spent. All the hip and elbow pillows were eliminated with the use of my new mattress, and we found that I rarely needed any adjusting during the night.

I had been home about two weeks when we had to reverse our nights and days in the iron lung, for I was out capacity time for daylight hours. Instead of sleeping all night in the respirator and staying in bed all day, I began sleeping in my bed at night.

Our neighbor came over and helped Harry carry me from the respirator into bed the first night, and Harry got me all settled for the night and crawled in beside me. Then I started to fidget mentally. I was still awake at 11:30, voicing a few doubts to Harry as to whether I would be able to breathe all night long out of the respirator. The neighbors were all in bed and there was not anyone to help carry me back to the respirator if I had wanted to go back, although Harry could carry me alone in an emergency. He had carried me alone to the respirator the first day that I was home, just to make sure that he could if something should happen. I knew I could get back into the respirator if need be, but I was admitting to myself that it was much more comfortable when two people carried me.

Finally, after listening to me for a while, Harry said, "Jean, you know Ross will be home from work around 12:30 and if you're still jittery, then I'll call him and ask him to help carry you back to the respirator. But in the meantime, why in hell don't you just shut up and go to sleep!" That did it. I did just that. When I awoke the next morning, it was 7:30; I had slept soundly and was still breathing. That was the last doubt I ever had that I would not be able to breathe through the night.

Harry, and the woman who was helping us, carried me back to the respirator in the morning. I stayed in all that day and received my packs in the respirator. From then on, we started working my time out of the respirator backwards, so to speak. Each week, I went back into the respirator later and later in the morning. I continued that schedule until I was finally completely free of the iron lung.

When I came home from the hospital, I had been told that therapy from the Visiting Nurse Association was not available in the home for more than one day a week, at the most. We were confused about the therapy and about how often I would need it. We wanted to be sure that I was getting adequate treatment, but in view of my fears and troubles at the hospital, we were inclined to be cautious. We hoped to repair the psychological damage that had been done, for I had a real problem by that time. The fear was very genuine and I was trying hard to battle with it, for in reality I was quite ashamed of my fears. I had never been a whiner, and I felt that I was not acting quite adult.

Finally, a friend of mine located a chiropractor who had had physical therapy training and who was interested in taking my case. Dr. Mericas was a young doctor who had been in practice for some time in our locality. He came out and talked with us one evening, and we arranged for him to give me therapy treatments three times a week. He used much the same methods with which I had become familiar, along with an electrical sine treatment and the chiropractic neck and back adjustments.

It took Dr. Mericas a long time to gain my confidence, but I gradually relaxed and we were able to see improvement showing up slowly. We have always felt deeply indebted to Dr. Mericas for his understanding and perseverance toward helping me to acquire a new lease on life. It was not easy for him, and I know that he must have felt limited oftentimes due to our makeshift equipment at home. As time wore on and my psychological barrier gradually disintegrated, we began looking toward the possibility of my eventually going to Georgia Warm Springs Foundation for treatment.

I had a big battle to fight with myself, and I often got off track. I was determined, however, that I was going to make the most I could out of the life that I had left. The rest of my story concerns what I did, and how. My husband, my daughter, and I are proud of the normalcy we have accomplished in our everyday living. We three have worked hard at it with lots of cooperation from our folks, our friends, and our neighbors, but every bit of effort put forth has been worthwhile.

CHAPTER 10

Problems Work Out

E ach day after I came home from the hospital brought to light at least one new situation for all of us to cope with. First, we discovered that we had various cooking and eating problems. Breakfast had never been a very interesting meal to me, so juice and coffee were about all I ever wanted. Harry usually fixed his own breakfast, and since Kris was not yet in school, our help usually fixed her breakfast when she arrived.

At this time, I could not feed myself at all, even when I was not encased in the iron lung. I do not think I had been bothered by having to be fed at the hospital. However, after I got home, there seemed to be something about being in my own house and having to be fed every bite of food that bothered me a great deal. It was not long until I was not eating much lunch, either. Dinnertime did not bother me as much as the other meals, because Harry fed me from his plate and we went right along talking and eating. He developed such a knack of doing it that neither of us was conscious of his having to feed me.

For the first month I was home, our suppers consisted mainly of rare steak, a big green salad, and a vegetable. I could not seem to get enough of salads and green vegetables. Since steak was unheard of in the hospital, I truly enjoyed that. My taste for steak, salad, and vegetables seemed to be almost a craving. It was expensive, but it probably did a lot toward making me stronger because I had eaten very little all the time I was in the hospital.

We decided that a backrest might help with my eating problem, so we bought one that was constructed like a deck chair. It has worked out so successfully that I am still using it to this day. The back reclined just enough that I was much more comfortable breathing than when I was sitting upright in a chair, and it gave me the feeling that I was almost normal. This feeling caused many tears to flow for a while because while in that position, I was almost sure that I could feed myself. It was very frustrating to try so hard and find that the fork just would not reach my mouth, and my hands trembled so that it was a struggle to get something on the fork to begin with.

Despite all my frustrations, we managed very well with our eating problem. It soon became second nature with Harry, because he had to feed me for a good eight months after I came home from the hospital. I eventually learned to feed myself lying down with just a pillow under my head and the plate propped almost under my chin. This accomplishment came long before I mastered the art of feeding myself on the backrest.

One morning, after I had been home approximately six weeks, my folks came to see me shortly after I had been taken out of the respirator. I was sitting in a chair in the living room when all of a sudden, I discovered that I could raise the lower portion of my right arm. It came out of the clear blue sky and I plainly remember how thrilled we all were with my accomplishment. I was always trying to do something I felt I could do but I was so amazed when it just happened, that I could scarcely speak.

What actually happened was that the muscles in that portion of my arm had gradually become stronger but had gone unnoticed by all of us until that very moment. This accomplishment eventually enabled me to feed myself while on the back-rest.

The woman who helped us left at four each afternoon, which left Kris and me alone until Harry came home some time between five and six. One of my neighbor-friends came over to stay with us during those hours for a month or so until her expected baby was born. After that, her thirteen-year-old daughter, Darlene, and Darlene's friend, Suzanne, took turns coming in after school and staying until Harry arrived at home.

Prior to this time, Harry had been preparing our supper after he got home from work. But after the girls had been coming in for a while, we decided that perhaps we could help Harry a little by getting supper started at least. Since we had been using a card table set up in the bedroom as our dinner table, the girls would begin by setting that up. Then, they would bring ingredients for simple casserole dishes or salads, and with my guidance, they always did a good job of getting our supper well underway. Both girls were used to helping their mothers at home, so they were quite capable, as well as willing.

It soon became interesting and helpful for me to give a little thought to what I could plan for the girls to get started the next week. This was really the beginning of the gradual return of my interest in housekeeping, and I began to feel that I was once again a part of the household. I had promised myself when I knew that I was leaving the hospital, that no matter how upset the house became, or how much I could see to be done, I was not going to voice any criticisms or let it bother me in any way. It just was not my nature not to take part in things, though, as this project with the two girls proved. I hope that I can do as fine a job raising my daughter as Darlene's and Suzanne's mothers did with them. It is very unusual to find two girls that age who are as dependable and as willing as Darlene and Suzanne were. I feel that they did a lot toward my rehabilitation by being so cooperative. The girls were excellent with Kris, too, and she not only enjoyed them but also learned a lot from them.

One of the things that I found most difficult to accept was that of not being mistress in my own home. For instance, I resented the fact that, whenever I wanted to see a particular item of correspondence, I would have to ask someone to go into our personal belongings to find it for me. It also bothered me to have someone bring the mail to me and leaf through it to tell me what was there, although she probably thought it was a big help to me. I was not ready to share my personal life with anyone at that time, and I finally got to the point where I never attempted to look at mail until Harry came home. I knew I was still unusually sensitive and time would help. I was learning that adjusting took lots of time, but we worked out a more tolerant attitude as I gradually did make necessary adjustments.

We had a woman come in on Saturdays to do scrubbing and give the house a good cleaning. My mother took over Kris' laundry and the rest of our laundry was sent out, so we did not have any ironing to be done at home. We found many shortcuts to keeping our housework to a minimum. For instance, since our floors were bare from necessity, we had our floors sanded throughout the house and a wax put on instead of varnish. This made a very attractive floor and one that was very easy to keep clean with a minimum amount of effort. We found that a little hard wax on steel wool would take up any number of black spots that were made by the respirator.

The day of the floor sanding resembled a three-ring circus while it lasted, but it was well worth it. I had a neighbor who had offered to come in and help during the day because everything had to be taken out of the closets and put back. The sanders started in the bedroom while I stayed in the respirator in the living room. Various boxes were removed from the bedroom closets and somehow managed to be put out on the front porch. It was not long before one of the children came in to tell us that our boxes were flying down the street. My neighbor had quite a time rescuing them.

When the men got out to the living room and worked around the respirator as well as they could, we asked one of them to help carry me back to the bedroom. It was always interesting to watch a stranger's face when asked to help carry me. I guess he was afraid that he was going to hurt me. Any stranger who was around me for any length of time was always surprised to discover that I did not hurt anywhere and that I did not feel sick.

I was truly a poor advertisement for polio, because I had so few muscles that had returned. However, I think people who met me understood better what polio is all about. It is surprising to discover some of the ideas that exist in the minds of some people about polio. For instance, we had some new neighbors move in across the street from us, and Harry offered to drive the woman of the house downtown one day when he happened to be going that way. He invited her to come over and visit us, and he mentioned that I had had polio. She told Harry that she had heard about me, and she wanted to tell him frankly that she was afraid to come over to see me because she was afraid she would get polio.

Harry explained to her that I had spent six months in the hospital and had been home several months, that our little girl had been accepted for school, and that he was sure that if there were any chance of contagion, I would not have been allowed to come home. She came over to visit me shortly after that, so I brought the subject up with her and we had a nice chat. I hope that I helped her understand polio a little more clearly, because it was obvious that it was a genuine fear with her.

I could very easily understand my neighbor's fear of polio, for I had grown up with that fear. My mother had always been extremely frightened of the disease. We had a neighbor boy who contracted it when he was at summer camp, and I remember what a tragedy it was in the neighborhood. That boy came out of his polio attack about 90 percent better than I did, but it was still a tragedy. He has a decided limp but gets along without even a cane. My mother never would let me go swimming when the summer's heat was at its worst, or when any specific warnings had been given regarding polio. My mother was a graduate nurse and was always extremely clean. Perhaps she kept me too well protected from germs. At any rate, it took me until I was almost thirty years old to pick up the poliovirus.

My mother had the same protective feeling for Kristin after she was born. I remember the year that we got polio I had mentioned taking Kris to a circus that was in town, and my mother discouraged it because she had read where the same circus had passed through a polio epidemic area. We did not go to the circus, but we both did get polio.

CHAPTER 11

More New Experiences

A fter I had been home a couple of months, we began to wonder how the summer was going to treat me, since I was flat on my back in bed most of the time. We decided that a sun porch might be helpful in keeping me comfortable throughout the summer months. We had a room, approximately 8' by 10' with seven windows and a door, built on the back of our house. This was one of the most worthwhile investments we ever made. We bought a studio couch for the room, and on the days when I did not get physical therapy treatment, Harry would carry me out to the porch in the morning before he left for work. It was a very pleasant place to be, for I could be put on the backrest so that I could see out the windows. Children came in and out often, which helped to pass the time pleasantly.

I learned that I could read pocket editions of books by tearing out a page at a time from the book. I still did not have enough strength in my hands to hold even a pocket-sized book. Harry would tear the covers off each book, which loosened the binding so that all I had to do was lift each page out. I was still reading in this manner when I went to Warm Springs in October of 1949, but I was not there very long before I was able to hold the book itself. This made more than one of us happy, for my method of reading with pages fluttering all over the floor did not make me a very welcome visitor as far as the attendants were concerned.

The longer I was home, the more I felt that I should be making an effort to sit up more often. Since I still had so much trouble breathing, we thought perhaps part of my trouble was not having a wheelchair in which to sit. I called the Foundation and asked about borrowing a wheelchair.

The chair arrived within a few days, and I was very anxious to try it. When I looked at it, though, I noticed with concern that it had springs under the seat. Springs ordinarily would not frighten anyone, but the first time I was lifted into that chair and those springs started to bounce I had visions of being picked up off the floor. I was aware of the fact that I was not about to do much moving around, but I was hard to convince that I was not going to fall out of the chair. Every time I as much as turned my head, I could feel the chair rock. It was like being sentenced to the guillotine every time I was put in it, so I finally gave up and sent the chair back.

The next time I was in a wheelchair was about a year later when Harry's cousin was married. She had asked Kris to be a flower girl at the wedding. My mother made Kris an adorable blue gown, and I was determined that I was going to go to the wedding.

We rented a portable wheelchair, hoping that I would be able to sit in it long enough to see the ceremony. The chair was delivered too late on the day of the wedding for me to try it out, so along with many other last minute preparations, the chair was tossed in the car, and we were ready to start.

Our friend and neighbor, Ross Holland, went to the wedding with us to help Harry get me in and out of the car. It was always easier to pick me up to put me into the car from a sitting position, rather than the prone position in which I was usually carried. Consequently, whenever I went out in the car, I was always carried to a chair close to the door and seated in that. Then, whoever was carrying me picked me up from the chair in a sitting position.

In our big rush that evening, Ross and Harry picked me up from the wrong side, and they got out to the car with me before discovering their mistake. My quick-thinking husband hung onto the upper part of me, slid into the car with me on his lap, and then had to slide out from under me. Believe me, he had to do it very fast, or I would have hollered bloody murder for fear that I was going to fall. Well, anyway, we were off to the wedding.

We wanted to be the last guests to arrive, but we had not intended to be as late as we were, for the music had already started. The boys decided that, instead of setting me up in the wheelchair outside, they would carry me into the vestibule of the church and set me up there to be sure that I did not miss the wedding. Away we went into the church.

We all got inside, with Harry and Ross carrying me, and they found they had forgotten to bring the wheelchair in before carrying me in. There was nothing to do but set me down on a wooden pew in the vestibule while one of them went back after the wheelchair. I was so thin that every bone in my body seemed to be sticking out through my skin and rubbing against that straight up and down, hard wooden pew. I was sure also that I was going to fall, and I was very unhappy, to say the least. The wedding party was standing out in the vestibule and they were probably nervous enough as it was without the to do I was putting on out there. Harry has always said that on that day, he knew that I would never walk again. I was so mad that he knew if I could have gotten up, that would have been the time. However, the worst was yet to come.

We got the wheelchair set up with me in it, and then we found out that the chair had a low back on it and did not give my back enough support to enable me to hold my head steady. I felt like I was going over backwards. Therefore, during the wedding and when we were greeting relatives, we tried to camouflage the situation with Harry standing behind me with my head resting against his stomach. It was quite a disappointment to me that I was not more comfortable in the wheelchair.

I thought so much about the wheelchair after we got home, that the next morning I asked Harry if he would try me in it once more. We had had company over the weekend, so Bob and Harry lifted me into chair once more. Once more, the tears started to flow when I thought Harry had let go of me and I thought I was falling. Harry reassured me, though, and I sat up for about a half-hour. It was a very tiring experience, for it was such a struggle for me to hold my back and neck steady. We have some moving pictures that were taken that Sunday, and I find it very amusing to look at them now. My eyes were as big as saucers, and the pictures would leave no doubt in anyone's mind that I was not exactly at ease.

The first and only trip that I ever made into Dr. Mericas' office must have been a sight to behold. The doctor felt that if I were put on a regular chiropractic adjusting table, he might be able to get better results from the therapy. I was frightened, but I thought that I should at least try to go.

I had Harry bring down one of my favorite skirts and a blouse, and since it was warm weather, I thought I would not bother with hose. I really felt quite festive when I was all dressed.

My dad decided to come along to help, so he and Harry got me into the car. While I was nervous about the whole thing, I was doing fairly well. That is until the car turned a corner and I happened to look down and I got a good look at my legs. It was the first time that I realized that my legs had become atrophied. It was not extensive but extremely noticeable to me. The fact that I did not have hose on and I had on black suede shoes did not help any. The atrophy had taken away the calves of my legs, and they looked straight up and down in back.

Until that day, I had always seen my legs stretched straight up ahead of me during my therapy treatments, and from the front, they looked just fine. It was quite a shock to discover that my legs had lost their shape, and it was a bitter blow to my vanity. My husband is no different from most men, and he had always had many comments to make regarding girls' legs. I knew then that mine were beyond causing any favorable comment. Tears still came readily those days, and I was a disheartened girl when we pulled up in front of the doctor's office.

Harry and my father got me into the office just fine. Dr. Mericas gave me an electrical spine treatment, I was quite comfortable, and the visit so far had been a success. After the electrical treatment, Harry and the doctor picked me up and started to put me on the adjusting table. The table was narrow, and they did not have a place, such as a cot or a stretcher, on which they could put me down and then roll me onto the table. They tried to put me down and turn me at the same time.

They succeeded, but they also succeeded in frightening me beyond description. When they turned me, they apparently stretched my body, and the pain combined with the fear of falling was a terrific experience. It was one time when I really screamed and cried, and no doubt swore.

It was a good thing that the visit has been pre-arranged and there were not any other patients in the waiting room, for I really put on a performance. It was worse than taking a child to the doctor. I screamed at both Harry and the doctor, and I am sure I would have kicked them both had I been able to move. I do not know how I got home except that I cried all the way. It was a very wearing experience for everyone, and one that we have never duplicated. When we look back on it now, it is very funny to all of us.

We kept the iron lung at our house for six to eight weeks after I was really out of it for good. I kept it the first few weeks for the feeling of safety it gave me, and the next couple of weeks, we were just waiting for someone from the Foundation to come and pick it up.

The respirator had been gone just a few days when I got an accumulation of phlegm in my throat because of a sinus attack or a cold—I do not remember which. I have always been bothered with chronic sinus plus a few allergies, and somehow or another, I got this accumulation in my throat. It rattled and I could not get it up or down. In trying to raise it, I became very tired. Consequently, I became panicky and this gave me a feeling of nausea. Finally, we called the doctor, and he came out and gave me a hypodermic, probably more to quiet me than for any other reason. Dr. Mericas also came out and administered artificial respiration for a while. I gradually was quieted down and I was able to get the phlegm loosed. That was the beginning of several such attacks.

I had one other very bad one a couple of months later. I had been sitting on the backrest on the porch. I knew I was going to have trouble before Harry left in the morning, but he was in a hurry that morning so I did not mention it. I became interested in watching the children playing outside, and I sat up on the backrest considerably longer than I should have, knowing that I did have the phlegm accumulation and could not possibly raise it when I was sitting up.

When I did lie down, I had such an accumulation that I found it hard to get my breath and I seemed to be choking. I was alone with the housekeeper, and I told her to call Dr. Mericas. She started to give me the phone, but all I could do was shake my head "no," and try to make her understand that she would have to do the talking. She finally got Dr. Mericas on the phone, told him who she was, and then shocked me when I heard her say, "Miss Denecke is not feeling very well and would like to have you come out."

I managed to get my voice enough to tell her to tell him I was choking, and I guess he understood since he made it out in record time. He relaxed me a little with some artificial respiration, and then he talked me into letting him carry me back to the bedroom where he could turn me over on my stomach. I was quite panicky and so scared that I would not get my next breath; I was ready to try anything. I had always been reluctant to be turned on my stomach during an attack because I felt smothered. This time, however, I was willing to do as he suggested.

As soon as the doctor turned me on my stomach, the blocked phlegm loosened and I was able to clear it. It was the most wonderful feeling that I have ever had, after struggling so long for air. Those attacks took a lot out of me, and I was always very weak and tired after them. They gradually diminished, and as I got stronger, I finally developed a feeling of confidence and knew that I could handle them. I was less panicky with each attack, and I won half the battle when I got over that terrific fear.

Getting back to my original statement about the iron lung—I just knew with the trouble I was having, that I would surely need the respirator again. I asked if they would get it back for me. It was not necessary, of course, and when I calmed down, I knew that I was going to be all right. However, those attacks were very vivid, and I do not know what caused them. I still have them occasionally on very hot, humid days, and always when I have a cold.

I guess a woman who has been ill is beginning to recuperate when she starts to think about her appearance. My particular concern all my life has been my hair. It is black, straight hair, very thick, and grows very rapidly. I had been wearing a feather bob when I got polio and had had a fresh permanent, but with the green soap shampoos that it had been getting and my poor diet, my hair was badly in need of attention.

Two of my friends volunteered to come out and at least give me a haircut. One of the girls had been a beauty operator and she was willing to tackle the job, so Betty and Harry lifted me into a chair and Lucille tried to style my hair. My neck was very wobbly, and every time the comb went through my hair, my head went right along with it.

I was having a great deal of difficulty breathing and it was a terrific struggle, so we finally decided that I just was not flexible enough to do a professional job. We were trying to change the style, but it was not too successful. I was certainly more comfortable with the shorter hair than I had been before, but there was not much curl left and I am afraid no efforts did much to improve my appearance.

My hair was washed at least every two weeks, and while it was easy to do, it involved a lot of time. To wash my hair, they used to put a rubber sheet under my head and towels around my shoulders. They then folded the rubber sheet into a funnel shape that led into a bucket on the floor. We used the teakettle to wet my head, and of course, it was easier when done by two people. There were many trips back and forth to empty the bucket and fill the teakettle. Harry had bought a hair dryer for me while I was in the hospital, for there was not one available there and I thought it was conducive to colds to lie with a damp head.

I had one professional haircut before I went to Warm Springs. When the definite date was made for me to go, I called the beauty shop where I had had my last permanent and asked if anyone ever came out from the beauty salon to the home. This began my association with Miss Johnson who has given me more than one morale boost with her haircuts and permanents.

It was always a struggle for anyone to work on my hair during those first two years of my illness, because I could not sit up long enough to get a complete permanent wave. Part of it had to be done while I was lying down and the rest while I was sitting up. I think Miss Johnson gave me two permanents in this awkward fashion.

11 - More New Experiences

While I was at Warm Springs, I had my hair cut shorter, and I decided that I looked better with the shorter style. After I came home from Warm Springs, my hair was again in need of attention, so I called Miss Johnson. The condition of my hair was greatly improved because I sat up in a wheelchair often, where previously my time in the chair had been very limited.

Miss Johnson decided that if I would wear a short haircut shaped and slightly shingled at the back with bangs and just a little curl around the face, I would be able to get by without a permanent. I have worn my hair in a similar fashion every since, and it is certainly a big help not to have to bother with permanents. It is also much more comfortable when I am lying in bed.

I have always been fortunate enough to have someone who is willing to do my hair once a week. Harry can even do it if necessary. Miss Johnson advised us on the type of scissors to buy, and Harry has learned to keep my hair trimmed in between haircuts.

Our first housekeeper stayed with us for a year. After she left, I was able to get help to take care of me and do more housework and cooking, because I did not require nearly the care that I did when I first came home. We have had any number of people working for us in the past five years. Some have been good, some have been bad, and some have been just downright impossible. Through it all, though, most of them have had their bad qualities.

Up until the time I went to Warm Springs, I had to give all of my directions from my bed, and when I was up, I was in one spot and had to stay there. However, when I was being carried I developed the habit of looking around, and Harry used to tell me I could see more when I was passing from room to room in those few seconds than most people saw when sitting and looking at something closely. Kris learned that I had extremely good ears, and it never ceased to amaze her how I knew she was

Walking Isn't Everything

into something and could tell her into what she was. The same thing was true for our hired help. I developed hearing so keen that I could tell what speed was being used on our electric stove. This habit had its points—both good and bad.

About the time we acquired our new housekeeper, I was trying to work out an arrangement of part-time cooking, nursing, and cleaning to everyone's satisfaction, we acquired a new cocker spaniel. I have always been very fond of dogs, and my sister-in-law gave us Spook when she found she could not take care of her and teach school at the same time.

Spook was approximately seven months old when we acquired her, and she was as impish and as cute a little black cocker as could be. She could run like greased lightning, and it was funny to hear Fanny Mae the housekeeper call Spook and forget to shut the door into the main part of the house. Spook would run right past Fanny Mae with her muddy feet, with Fanny Mae in close pursuit shooing her apron and clucking at the pup at the same time. By that time, Spook would be up on the bed on top of me—mud and all—with my older cocker spaniel following suit. I loved both of them, but I am sure they were not much help to the sheet situation, or the help situation, either.

Mandy, the older cocker spaniel, acquired a fungus infection and many people told me that she would never get over it. Mandy had been my pet since the year before Kris was born and I was determined that she was going to be cured. She had always been a very healthy dog, and I think diet negligence on our part in adjusting to my coming home made her susceptible to the fungus.

We tried everything on her, but nothing seemed to help much. She was down almost to bare skin, and that is losing a lot of hair for a cocker spaniel. She came through it just fine after many months, but eventually Spook got the fungus from Mandy.

While I was in Warm Springs, Spook got so bad that the veterinarian advised Harry to have her put to sleep. She had a much more excitable disposition than our older cocker, and I think the constant itching had bothered her a lot more than it had Mandy.

Kris and I would like to have two dogs again some day, but neither of us has the nerve to insist.

Walking Isn't Everything

CHAPTER 12

Off to Warm Springs

My first year at home from the hospital passed very rapidly, and with each passing day, I found that my outlook improved. We began to talk about and think seriously about the possibility of my going to the Georgia Warm Springs Foundation for treatment.

We were still very hopeful that I would some day walk again, but there were times when my spirits were low. When this happened, I would always start to cry, and I told Harry that I did not want to wear braces and struggle to walk. As time went on, though, these periods of depression came less often.

I often think back to some of my ideas in early polio, especially when some of my friends from Warm Springs who use braces and crutches as aids in walking are around. Before I became educated in handicap aids, I visualized braces as being strapped on the outside for everyone to see. In reality, braces are very artfully designed so clothing can easily camouflage them.

I am relating my thoughts as I remember them, because I think they are typical of the thoughts that one has in early polio, but they are thoughts of ignorance, even though one is an adult. You just cannot quite make up your mind that you are ready to accept a half-way measure, either. Your thoughts at this time are so confused that they can be compared to the difference between adult thinking and childhood thinking.

To anyone reading this who might be in the early stages of polio, I would like to say that all these mixed-up feelings have a way of working out, and it is not too long until you are able to look back and laugh at some of the ideas that you had. After being around handicapped people, you forget the aids they use, because the result is so gratifying.

The first fall I was home, Kris started to school and the privilege of going with her fell to Daddy instead of Mother. I later became acquainted with her teacher over the telephone, and once again, we were fortunate because our child liked school. She also liked her teacher, so our telephone acquaintance was adequate and satisfactory.

Christmas that year came and went, and Christmas morning found me sitting out in the living room bright and early as Kris opened her presents. It was fun for me, and still another important step toward normalcy in our family life.

In the spring of 1948, a columnist for one of the local papers sponsored a drive for funds to purchase a television set for the polio patients at the hospital to which I had been confined for the first six months of my illness. I was extremely anxious to help, so I interested my two friends, Darlene and Suzanne, and their girlfriends in having an ice cream festival in our backyard.

The idea met with great enthusiasm, and our neighbor told me of a friend of hers on the next street who worked for a creamery. She suggested that he might be able to get us a discount on Dixie cups. I contacted this man and told him of our plans. He was so enthusiastic that when he told his fellow workers about it, they not only bought the Dixie cups for us but also started our fund off with $10.00.

On the day of the festival, the girls carried a picnic table and benches over from Suzanne's house and put them in our backyard. I bought some crepe paper that the girls used to decorate the table and the yard, and the scene was very festive looking. The kids made cardboard signs, put them in a couple of the local store windows, and tacked them up around the house a few days in advance.

The weather was just perfect on the day of the festival. Harry carried me out to the back porch and put me up on the backrest where I could see all the activity. The neighborhood turned out en masse, along with quite a few friends whom I had called, and everything went off beautifully. Our cookies had been donated as well as the ice cream, so when the festival was over and the receipts counted, we found that we had over $40.00—all clear profit for the television fund.

The next day was Saturday, and Harry took the girls down to the newspaper office with the money. Our young daughter went with them. She had been all decked out like the big girls at the party. When the girls presented the money, they told their story of the festival, and the news staff took a picture of the group. The picture appeared in the paper a couple of days later, and of course, all the girls were duly thrilled by it.

I was becoming very anxious to go to Warm Springs, for a friend of ours, who had been a patient there numerous times, had told me a lot about it. Ann had had polio when she was fifteen years old, and she had been given a very dark outlook as to her chances for recovery. After having had polio for more than a year, she had been sent to Warm Springs for treatment, and she now does a beautiful job of walking. She had enough good muscles that they were able to help her with surgery. She walks well enough to be able to hold an excellent position at a popular restaurant in western Michigan, and she spends a good share of the day on her feet.

Walking Isn't Everything

Ann came to see me when I was in the hospital, and she encouraged me a great deal by telling me all about Warm Springs. I was very enthusiastic about going while I was still an early patient at the hospital. However, I could not go then because of the iron lung, and later, I just was not interested in going back to any hospital. The desire to go to Warm Springs was in the back of my mind, though, and all I needed was the courage so say that I would go.

Harry was badly in need of a vacation away from the monotony of being limited in activities and caring for me, so I suggested that perhaps he might go down to Warm Springs to see what it was like. It happened that Ann was making one of her frequent visits at the same time, so she showed him all around the hospital. He came home very enthusiastic about what he had seen. We decided then that it was time for me to make the trip.

The first thing I had to do before I could go to Warm Springs was to find a suitable housekeeper to take care of Kris, since my mother was no longer able to do it. Mother had had major surgery performed the first fall I was home, and she was a long time recuperating. She would have made the effort to care for Kris, but Kris had started to school and we felt that she was old enough then to be left with some competent person so that it would not be another complete uprooting for her.

It took quite a while to find the right person. I tried advertising, but I finally found a very capable person through an acquaintance. After I did find her, she was very patient in waiting for me to be straightened around and to get the admitting date from Warm Springs.

I really had a busy time before I got myself off on the trip. I wanted to be sure that so many things were taken care of before I left. From the preparations being made for my pending departure, I am sure that anyone who had been listening would have thought that I was not expecting to come back home.

12 - Off to Warm Springs

Our house was overflowing the week I left. My friend Marguerite, who is a nurse, offered to go with us, so she and her husband came up several days before we were to leave, to get my clothes and everything in order. Miss Rene, the housekeeper, came several days before we left, too, to be familiar with everything and to get to know Kris. My mother came out every day around noon and stayed until evening.

During that week, we were all trying to eat in the bedroom on the card table, and Fanny Mae was chief cook with a variety of assistants. Somehow or other we managed to get through the week, even though the evening before we left found me soaking my feet in the living room when some last minute callers came. Marguerite had been giving me a pedicure. Our neighbors brought me a very nice manicure set in a black leather case, which was a lovely surprise. It turned out to be a very useful gift, not only at Warm Springs, but ever since.

The Foundation had called and said that they thought they would be able to make flying arrangements for the trip to Warm Springs with the National Guard. It seemed that some of the pilots at a local air base needed flying hours, and they were going to work out an arrangement with the National Foundation whereby they would fly polio patients to Atlanta. This was to be the first trip made under these arrangements, and we were scheduled to leave the air base at 6:00 A.M.

We decided that, since it was such an early morning take-off and it was chilly October weather, it would be best to have the ambulance take me out to the plane instead of riding in the car. We were very glad we made this decision, because the plane was not ready when we arrived, and it was cold. The man who owned the ambulance happened to be personally acquainted with the pilot, and he suggested that they just leave me on the ambulance cot for the trip. When the plane returned from Atlanta, the pilot could call and have the cot picked up. This was a wonderful arrangement as far as I was concerned, because

I did not get cold at all, and the cot was very comfortable. The plane had very few seats and it had been outfitted for ambulatory patients.

We got away from the air base about 7:00 A.M. on the big day. We landed at a nearby town to pick up two other patients who were also going to Warm Springs, along with some Foundation personnel. One of the patients was a woman about my age who was accompanied by her husband, and the other was a five-year-old girl accompanied by her mother. Photographers also boarded the plane there, and we got the usual publicity— "Off to Warm Springs."

We had a very nice trip and arrived in Atlanta early in the afternoon. Two ambulances from the hospital and two passenger cars met us. Marguerite and I shared one ambulance with Connie and her mother, while Virginia and her husband rode in the other. Harry rode with the remaining passengers in one of the passenger cars.

Warm Springs Foundation is about 75 miles from Atlanta. When we arrived there, the cot was lifted from the ambulance and I got my first glimpse of the hospital and surroundings. I was wheeled past a very well groomed, middle-aged man in a wheelchair. He gave me a big smile and said, "I can sure tell you're an old timer." I thought to myself that he must be Mr. Fred Botts, the registrar at Warm Springs, who is himself a polio and is more or less an institution around the hospital. I was flattered by his greeting, and his remark proved to me that I had had polio long enough that I did not look sick and I was able to have a ready smile on my face.

CHAPTER 13

Georgia Warm Springs Foundation

C onnie, the little girl who had been on the same plane I was on to Warm Springs, was admitted to the children's ward after we arrived at the Foundation. Virginia was taken to the medical building, and I was sent to the second floor of the East Wing.

Being an old hand at rapid observation, I took in much as I was wheeled up to my room. I went past a couple of therapy rooms and some of the bedrooms. Some rooms had wheelchairs with odd-looking rods sticking up over the tops of them, and I saw crutches or braces stacked in corners.

There was not the usual medicinal odor of a hospital, but there was a familiar odor of steam because of various types of moist heat therapy used in the treatment rooms. I later learned that most of the rooms were two-bed rooms, and there were a few single rooms as well as a few with four beds in them.

Each room had its own washbowl, double closet, a dresser, and a nightstand for each patient. The rooms were quite spacious with tile floors and big windows. The dressers were varnished and quite beaten up along the bottom where patients, who could not reach over to shut a drawer, more often than not found a way to kick it shut or push it shut with a crutch. I am afraid that no one was very careful of furniture at Warm Springs, but the whole atmosphere was like a nice, comfortable, and well lived in house.

The halls were spacious and there was always a lot of activity—never an atmosphere of quietness that you find in an ordinary hospital. There was always lots of conversation with wheelchairs going this way and that, stretchers being wheeled up and down the halls, and much free visiting in rooms after treatment hours. I had been assigned to a two-bed room, and I was glad when I observed that my bed was the one next to the windows. Looking out windows had become an important pastime to me in the two years that I had lived with polio.

Marguerite helped the attendant get me settled in bed. The attendant asked me if I could feed myself, and that was the only question asked of me—none of the usual hospital routine as to history. We had a delicious supper that night. In fact, every meal served at Warm Springs while I was there was equal to that of a first-class restaurant. Fried chicken was frequently on the menu, and we always had homemade hot rolls.

Some patients had to be on a low-calorie diet, so with such wonderful menus, it was no wonder that moans and groans were heard from the low-calorie section. Excess weight can be very hindering to the functional ability of a polio, and sadly enough, the limited activity frequently leads to avoirdupois. I only had a few meals in the dining room, but I learned some of the routines, and I found out that they had a very nice arrangement for their low-calorie (LC) patients. All those who were LC patients sat in one section of the dining room. Saccharin was always placed on these tables, and by segregating them from patients who were not on LC diets, the temptation was not as great.

New patients are not allowed up until one of the medical staff checks them. Since I arrived on a Friday, I was not examined until Monday. However, I was allowed to be wheeled around the Foundation on a stretcher. Naturally, I had had no treatment prescribed, and Harry and Marguerite came and went as they pleased. Marguerite wore her uniform the next morning so that she could do private duty for me while she was there.

To get back to the day after we arrived at Warm Springs, Harry wheeled me around the Foundation, and we learned a few interesting items about the background of Georgia Warm Springs Foundation.

We knew that it was through the efforts of Franklin D. Roosevelt that the Warm Springs Foundation was incorporated in 1927 as a non-profit institution for the treatment of the aftereffects of infantile paralysis. I am going to try to paint a word picture of the campus, but I am sure that my efforts will be very meager in giving due justice to the beauty of the entire outlay.

The campus is shaped like a quadrangle, and consists of buildings named as follows: Georgia Hall, two dormitories— Kress Hall and Builders Hall, the playhouse, chapel, pool, brace shop, infirmary, medical building, East Wing, and the school and occupational therapy building. There are also thirty-six Foundation-owned cottages for the staff members.

Georgia Hall is colonial in design and the citizens of the State of Georgia bequeathed it to the Foundation. I would describe it as a huge sitting room, furnished with a television set, piano, writing desks, card tables, and many lounge chairs placed in friendly groupings. The admitting desk for check-up patients is at one end of the hall, as is a small variety store where Cokes, candy, magazines, and gift articles are sold. There are several entrances to Georgia Hall. The dormitory, Builders Hall, and the dining room both adjoin Georgia Hall.

The playhouse is a separate building and was created in 1935 by remodeling an old outdoor dance pavilion that was originally on the premises. It is here that patients see movies three times a week. The Chapel is a separate building also, having been built in 1937, and the sheer simplicity of design is inspiring.

Every building at the Foundation is colonnaded, so that patients can go from one building to another in all kinds of weather without getting wet. All the buildings are snowy white, and the landscaping and trees are exquisite. In front of the medical building is a concrete area known as the walking court. When patients are ready for that particular therapy, they are walked twice a day, always with therapists' supervision. There are three sets of parallel bars of graduated sizes to assist patients in standing. There is also a platform of steps for practice.

Another building is known as the school and occupational therapy building. In it are classrooms, a library, and a craft shop that a large majority of the patients in residence frequent.

East Wing has an upstairs porch and a downstairs porch, and the medical building has balcony porches that make it easy for patients to be moved out into the sun in their beds. The lower floor of the medical building houses the surgical and administrative departments. The building that houses the pool has several treatment rooms, as well as dressing rooms, in conjunction with it.

The unique manner in which patients are transported from one building to another is interesting. It works like a taxi service, except that the patient supplies the vehicle and all that is called for is a driver. The drivers are called "push boys." These push boys operate from a station at the pool until 4:00 P.M., and then they operate from the front desk in Georgia Hall. Although the pool station is the main one, others operate during the day.

Push boys are assigned to a station, and they are directly responsible for transporting patients to and from the therapy or activity to which their station is assigned during treatment hours. Push boys are always available until bedtime and will take you anywhere on the campus.

The push boy system is excellent, because it enables all patients, not just those who are able to wheel themselves, to get about. I cannot say enough good things about whoever had the forethought to adopt the idea.

Patients for whom hydrotherapy has been prescribed are wheeled to the pool right in their stretchers even though they are not in wheelchairs. The push boy calls for the patient at the room with a stretcher, picks the patient up, lays him on the stretcher, and wheels him to the pool. The patient has been dressed in a bathing suit by an attendant or himself, if he is able, and is, of course, always supposed to be ready when the push boy arrives. The stretcher is wheeled into the room where the pool is, and the patient lies on the stretcher until the therapist is ready to start the treatment. The push boy leaves, taking any patient, who has had his therapy and is ready to return, back to his room. Then he brings another patient back to the pool on his return trip. He continues this shuttle all during treatment hours if this happens to be his assignment.

When the therapist is ready to begin treatment, two push boys in bathing suits, who do nothing but lift patients in and out of the water, lift you from your stretcher into the arms of your therapist. She in turn tows you to a table or chair in the water where you will have your therapy that day.

The therapist has no trouble towing a patient in the water. Many people have the mistaken idea that the springs at the Foundation have some magic power to heal, which is not true at all. It is just that the springs are natural, and the temperature and water combination are ideal for exercising weakened parts of the body.

Walking Isn't Everything

Kress Hall is a dormitory, and when I was a patient at Warm Springs, it was used mainly for lodging check-up patients. It too had a large lounge room and it was frequently used for various club meetings.

The brace shop is set back of the pool on a little dirt road, and I understand its original size has been doubled. The brace shop is just what its name implies——a building where appliances are made according to doctors' prescriptions, fitted, and adjusted.

It was still nice and warm in October when I arrived at Warm Springs, so we were able to spend a big part of Saturday outdoors. I was very favorably impressed with the campus grounds and the clean, white, well-designed buildings. However, the spirit of Warm Springs impressed me most of all. It is difficult to define this spirit, but the resort-like, college-like atmosphere, combined with the feeling of normalcy I had after arriving there, inspired new hope in me for physical and mental improvement.

One incident that Harry and I will always remember is a visit that a man we shall call Mr. Beal paid us the first evening we were there. This man was in his forties and had been a patient at Warm Springs for over a year. He was going home the next day, and that evening he was going up and down the hall saying his goodbyes. When he got to my room, he was wringing wet from the effort that he had had to make to walk. I want to say that I know from experience that walking after you have had polio is not just a matter of will power, no matter how many people tell you that if you have faith and determination you can walk. It just is not true. Mr. Beal had barely enough muscles to walk, and those that he did have were extremely weak. However, it was obvious that he was one of those few borderline cases who were walking from sheer determination. As I remember, the length of his stay at Warm Springs was the longest of any one patient.

My medical examination was scheduled for 1:00 on Monday afternoon, and I was full of butterflies from Sunday on. I was to be given a muscle test before the doctor's examination, so Marguerite accompanied me down to the examining room.

I am sorry to say that I had a very curt and unsympathetic therapist for my initial muscle test. However, it turned out to be one of the best things that happened to me while I was there, for it enabled me to become a patient of not only one of the best, but one of the sweetest therapists at the Foundation. I have stated before that I had very few muscles, my coordination was extremely poor, and I was scared to death, so maybe the combination of all this discouraged the therapist. I was still quite tight, and in the course of the examination, I was hurt and tears came to my eyes. Marguerite was very sympathetic and wiped at my eyes, which apparently did not meet with the therapist's approval. She told me that would not be the last time I was hurt in the next few months. In view of my experiences with therapy at the other hospital and the length of time it took me to make up my mind to go to Warm Springs, her reception certainly did not do anything to help matters.

After the therapist had finished the muscle test, the staff doctor came in and sat me up on the side of the stretcher. He looked me over, did a few superficial examinations, and then studied my muscle chart. I will always remember his first words to me after he had finished his examination. They were, "You know that there isn't a part of your body that hasn't been affected by polio, don't you?"

The doctor went on to tell me that I would never walk again. Strangely enough, this was not much of a shock, because it had been almost two years since I had become ill and we had suspected it for a long time. He looked at my hands and told me that there was quite a bit they could do to straighten them and increase their functional ability.

He recommended straight therapy with no hydrotherapy for the present, hot paraffin baths for my hands, heat applied to my shoulders if they were extremely tight, and a moderate amount of loosening. They did not like a patient with few muscles to become too loose, because you would be limp and resemble a rag doll. He did not recommend therapy on my legs. An orthopedic garment was to be ordered, and a portable wheelchair in due time. My hands were to be put in splints that he later specifically designed. I told him that my last vital capacity test had registered 850, and he said not to worry about that because it was considerably higher now.

The doctor had a very forthright way of speaking, and certainly, what he had to tell me was not spectacular or even very encouraging. Yet somehow, he had managed to encourage me a great deal, and I left his room with a good feeling. He told me that he thought I could be taught to turn myself over in bed, which made a big impression on me. I am sorry to say that it never materialized, though, try as hard as we could.

Harry was waiting in my room to hear what Marguerite and I had to say. When I told him what the doctor had said, I also told him about the therapist's reception, and in the back of my mind, I knew that the old fear had taken its hold on me again. In addition, although I did not admit it until later on in the evening, I wanted to go home.

I was upset the next day, for Marguerite had planned to go home that day. She was also unsettled in her mind as to whether it was the time to leave me. We both had heard so many wonderful reports about Warm Springs that frankly, we were both disappointed at the incident that we encountered with the therapist when I was given my muscle test. Marguerite decided when she came in the next morning and found me so upset that we would go over to see the head therapist to find out if she could help in any way.

Marguerite was extremely successful in her mission. She explained my history to the head therapist and told her that I wanted to go home. When Marguerite came back to my room, she told me that the head therapist would be over to see me. She came over shortly and I apologized to her for my tears. I explained that I had had polio long enough that I did not cry easily any more and that it was not my true nature to cry. I was ashamed of my fears. She appeared to understand, and she reassured me that if I would stay, she was confident that my therapy would not be too severe. She said she thought I would enjoy having Lynn Patten as my therapist. She was sure that Lynn would be very understanding, because she had an older brother who had polio the year before and who shortly would be a patient at Warm Springs himself.

The head therapist was successful in assuring me that my stay at Warm Springs would be pleasant, and that they could do a great deal for me. She was so helpful that Marguerite was able to leave that afternoon with a satisfied mind, and I was ready to start my therapy the next day.

Lynn Patten was everything and more that her superior had promised. She was about twenty-four years old—a real cute little black-haired girl with a marvelous sense of humor, and she was a very understanding, yet conscientious therapist. We became very good friends during my four-month sojourn at Warm Springs.

Lynn delights in telling people how big my eyes were when I was first wheeled into the treatment room. This is no exaggeration on her part, because I was by no means at ease. There was lots of activity in the treatment room— a patient on the table, one in the steamer, and I was pulled up alongside the paraffin vat. Lynn had been told of my burns and my sensitivity to heat, so she went very carefully with the paraffin. She too found that I burned very easily. Later on, when anyone complained that the paraffin bath was too hot, he or she was always told that if Jean Denecke could stand it, it was not too hot.

The hand was dipped three times in the liquid paraffin, which is kept at approximately 125 degrees. The actual dipping does not burn so much; it is when the hand is pulled out and cooled between each dipping that it really burns. You become accustomed to it, however, and the fingers are so much more flexible after the treatment. This makes your therapy less painful and you get to the point where you do not mind the paraffin dip at all.

Chemical heat was tried on my shoulders, but my shoulder burned so easily that they finally just put wet towels on my shoulders and turned on a heat lamp whenever heat was indicated to loosen my shoulders.

The therapy division where I had my treatment was located on the ground floor of East Wing, and push boy took patients to and from this activity, similar to the pool arrangement I have described. The therapy treatments lasted anywhere from one half-hour to an hour and were scheduled twice a day. The paraffin treatment was given only once a day, as was the treatment on my shoulders. The rest of my therapy involved stretching and muscle re-education.

After Marguerite left, Harry stayed with me the rest of the week. With him there to help lift me and wheel me around, we had a good week. We met other patients, and I began to adjust to the routine. Harry enjoyed himself, and he picked up quite a few ideas about equipment and methods of handling patients.

One of the most novel and interesting sights to watch was the way movie night was handled at Warm Springs. Movies are shown Monday and Wednesday evenings for adults, and there is a Saturday matinee for the children. The selection of pictures is excellent, so almost everyone goes to the movies.

Those patients who are not able to go to the movies in wheelchairs went right in their stretchers. Stretchers were put in the front of the playhouse, which was large enough for wheelchairs to be grouped back of the stretchers, and then there were the regular tiered seats for those who were not patients.

Movie night was really a busy night for push boys, attendants, and orderlies. There were usually enough stretchers to go around, but occasionally someone was left behind. In addition, some of the stretchers were more comfortable than others, so from the end of treatment time, when stretchers were no longer in use, there was a wild scramble when everyone spoke to his favorite orderly or attendant on the floor for a comfortable stretcher.

The stretcher was wheeled into the room, and several pillows were put under the mattress to raise it so that the patient was not lying perfectly flat. There was always lots of adjusting of pillows, for once you were in the movies it was hard to get attention, so it was important that you were settled comfortably before you set out. Sometimes, something started to hurt during the movie, though, and you ended up with tears rolling down your cheeks. However, it was dark and nobody could see. Besides, the movies were always good and worth the discomfort.

When you were settled on your stretcher about a half-hour before it was time for the movie to start, the push boys came up to the different floors and started making a line of stretchers in the hall until they had a long train. When they had quite a few lined up out in the hall, they started the train rolling by walking at the side of the stretchers, guiding and pushing at the same time until they reached the elevators. The train again lined up on the first floor as it came off the elevators, and when it was complete, it took off down the first floor hall and out the door onto a ramp leading into the playhouse. The same kind of train was made up of wheelchairs for those who had good arms and backs, enabling them to hold onto the chair in front of them.

This system required the help of only three or four push boys per train, so the playhouse was filled quite rapidly. Sometimes the speed of the train made you catch your breath, but it was always a hilarious ride with lots of singing and noise as the train rolled along.

By the time Harry left, I had made a few acquaintances, my therapy was coming along fine, and I seemed to be adjusting fairly well to the Foundation. Since he planned to leave early one morning, we said our goodbyes the night before. They were said without any qualms or hesitation on my part, for I had definitely made up my mind that I could be helped at Warm Springs, and that I was there to get the very most out of it that I possibly could.

The first roommate I had was an older woman, who had had unfortunate surgery done elsewhere and was a patient at Warm Springs for repair work. Her husband had accompanied her to the Foundation and stayed right with her, rooming in town. She was gone from the room a great deal, because patients who have had surgery and are in casts do not receive treatments during the period they are in casts. Naturally, such patients have a lot of free time, and since her husband was there to be a personal push boy, she spent very little time in the room. There were times when I wished I had a more compatible roommate.

During our tour of the buildings while Harry was still with me, we had talked with a very pleasant young girl on the first floor whose name was Charlotte Murphy. She told us that her husband was in the Air Force and that she had two children. Charlotte was a recent polio, and her involvement was not too extensive, most of it being in one leg and foot.

Patients are constantly being moved, some going to surgery, others being released. It was just a couple of weeks after I arrived that news got around that some moves were to be made. I was pleasantly surprised to find myself with Charlotte as a roommate. That was another of those wonderful breaks that came to me while I was at Warm Springs.

The fact that Charlotte was more AB (able-bodied) than I was and was so willing, at the same time, to help me was a big boost to my morale. She seemed to understand perfectly the little problems that bothered me a lot. I could not comb my own hair, and I never needed to ask Charlotte to do it for me. My nylon sweaters were always washed when she did hers. Since I could not wheel myself and my sitting up time was indeterminate, my activities would have been curtailed largely except for Charlotte. With her along when I went visiting, I knew I would never be stranded in someone's room. Sitting up for several hours is not a feat that comes to a polio without practice. Most of your padding is gone and you hope for calluses.

One of my ambitions was to go to the movies in my wheelchair instead of on a stretcher. Charlotte and I had discussed the possibility of it, and one evening we got brave and decided it could be done. We made one big mistake though when vanity got the best of me and I was decked out in new shoes. New shoes can get very uncomfortable, even on feet that do not move, so halfway through the picture, Charlotte had to remove one of my shoes, which was no easy task for her to perform on swollen feet from a sitting position.

My feet were not very hurt either, and before the movie was over, Charlotte was smoothing wrinkles from under me. We managed to stay for the complete movie, but the few remaining movies I saw before I was released were from a stretcher. In those days, I was still apprehensive of my endurance and I was probably expecting more trouble than I needed to.

Charlotte and I roomed together for four months, and we succeeded in establishing a completely harmonious relationship, sometimes under trying circumstances, too. Disappointments

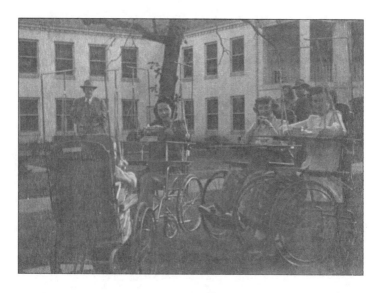

Jean Denecke with other patients at Warm Springs

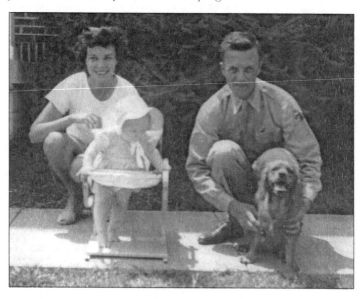

Jean, Kris, and Harry Denecke 1944

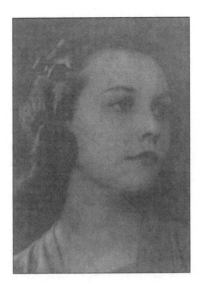

Jean Leeper as young woman

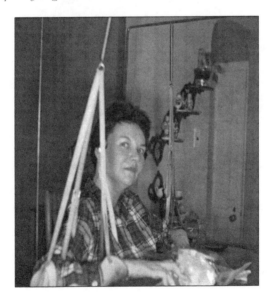

Jean Denecke at home in 1960's

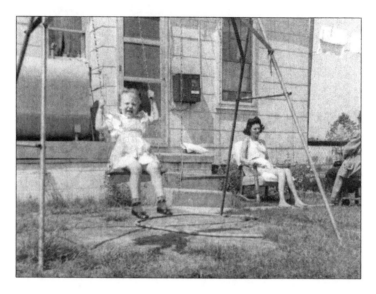

Jean Denecke with her mother and Kris before Warm Springs

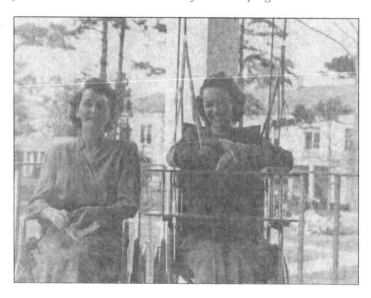

Jean Denecke with her roommate Charlotte at Warm Springs

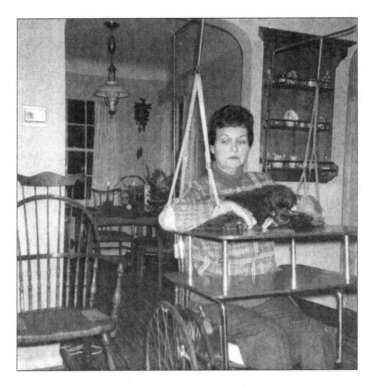

Jean Denecke with dog Henri on her lapboard. December 1963

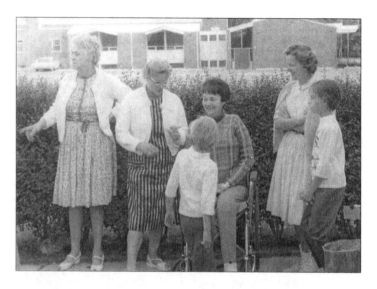

Jean Denecke at backyard party in 1960's

CHAPTER 14

Incomparable
Aids for Me

Within a couple of weeks after my treatments began, I was wheeled up to the corset shop to have measurements taken for my orthopedic garment. Nearly everyone—men, women, and children alike—wear these individually fitted orthopedic garments. Some patients dislike their corsets, and then again, there are patients like myself who are aided so tremendously by wearing one that they would not think of getting up without it.

Mine is particularly heavily stayed for support. Measurements are taken for the garment; you go back a week later for a fitting; and sometime during the following week, your corset is delivered to you and you begin wearing it. I had no difficulty at all in getting used to it. I have very weak abdominal muscles, so when I sat up before the time I was fitted with my corset, my stomach protruded and my innards seemed to drop, which was making it more difficult for me to breathe while sitting up. After putting on the corset and being strapped and laced into it firmly, I could breathe 75% better. I also found that I did not tire so easily.

Another physical aid I was learning to use were arm slings that had been fitted to my wheelchair. Arm slings are funny-looking, overhead upside down L-shaped rods that are attached to the back of the chair at each side. An ordinary screen door spring is slid onto each rod. From that spring, two leather straps are suspended with a cushioning on each—one for the elbow and one for the wrist. These straps can be adjusted to various heights and must never be pulled tight enough to hike a shoulder.

Along with this arm-sling equipment comes a lapboard—a board bringing things to a workable height in relation to the slings. The old-fashioned wooden wheelchairs, which were predominantly used at Warm Springs, had single lapboards that were attached to the chair and could be adjusted as to height. The portable chairs had double lapboards, which were slid onto the chair arms and were adjustable.

I remember how odd arms slings appeared to me the first time I saw them, and when I was first put into them, I could not see any earthly use for them except that the springs enabled you to jiggle your arms and swing them back and forth. When I tried to eat in them, I was extremely clumsy. In fact, everything that I tried to do while using them was very awkward at first.

Now, however, my arm slings, like my corset, are indispensable. They do many things for me that make me feel that I could not do without them. I am never without them when I am in my own home. For one thing, they aid my breathing by creating a weight balance. I have very few shoulder muscles, so in sitting in a chair without slings, the weight of my shoulders and arms becomes heavy on my respiratory muscles.

The slings also help me to balance my body, enabling me to use both hands. When I went to Warm Springs, I was not able to comb my own hair. As I progressed in using arm slings, my therapist and I learned that by adding extension handles to a small size brush and comb I could manage to comb all but a small portion of the back of my hair. The handles were designed and made at the brace shop, and my success in using them sold me 100% on arm slings. I used the extension handles for a few months after I came home, but as I got stronger, I found that I no longer required their assistance.

I have been amazed many times at the ease with which I can now do many things, such as write, sew, play cards, help with the cooking, eat, and drink. All credit must go to the Warm Springs arm slings for my ability to perform these operations.

Everyone goes to clinic once a month at Warm Springs, and in between times, if any new equipment has been issued to the patient. Dr. Bennett and Dr. Britt usually hold clinic one afternoon a week, with various therapy heads present. Each therapist takes her own patients in one at a time. The doctors check progress, equipment, etc., and additional orders are discussed and given at that time. Clinic visits afford the patient an opportunity to ask any questions he might have on his mind and time up is always granted at these visits. The patient, in receiving such intensified professional attention, experiences a feeling of confidence and progress.

After treatments were over for the day, which could easily be early in the afternoon, patients' time was their own. There were always card games and television at Georgia Hall, and lots of visiting went back and forth between rooms. An atmosphere of freedom was prevalent, because no one paid any attention to the comings and goings of patients at the Foundation itself, but a pass was required when leaving the premises.

It was not long until I was called to the brace shop to have measurements taken for hand splints. The splints were made of aluminum and Dr. Britt designed them to do the required straightening of my fingers. It took many fittings, plus many trips to clinic, before the splints were acceptable to Dr. Britt. They would be hard to describe, so I will not say any more except that I still use them and they have done a great deal to straighten my fingers, thus enabling me to use them to better advantage.

Every two months, each patient is given a muscle test to measure progress. After I had been at the Foundation several weeks and my treatments were progressing satisfactorily, I was given occupational therapy. I believe I had this two or three times a week. When my hand splints were designed, a special set was made for me to use during my occupational therapy treatments. This was my first experience with this type of treatment, and it was lots of fun as well as being beneficial.

Occupational therapy had many limitations, however, as I was concerned. There were many things that I just could not do, as well as lots of things that I should not do while my muscles were being re-educated. Paper and cloth stenciling were among the few activities that were enjoyable to me.

CHAPTER 15

Time Passes Quickly

The days passed quite rapidly at Warm Springs. The weather was a big help, because nearly all winter it was possible to sit out on the porches, wearing just a light sweater.

There was enough to do that time very seldom dragged. Treatments were omitted on Saturday afternoons, and that was when I usually had my hair done by one of my favorite attendants. She shampooed my hair first, putting me on a stretcher and wheeling me into the bathroom. My head was hung over the end of the stretcher and washed over the bathtub with a spray. Then there was plenty of time for an orderly to get me up in the wheelchair after the shampoo, so that the attendant could put my hair up in pins. Incidentally, a beauty shop was the one thing that was lacking at Warm Springs Foundation, although there was one in the town itself. Many of the girls are able to pin curl their own hair, and some are even able to shampoo it themselves. I was fortunate enough to find a young girl who would do mine for a nominal fee.

Every patient got a bath once a day. Some patients, such as my roommate, needed just a little assistance in getting into the tub, and then they bathed themselves. Two maids did nothing but give baths every morning to patients in my condition. A schedule was adhered to for baths, so that each patient got his bath at approximately the same time every morning. The maids wheeled the stretcher in, rolled you onto it, and the two of them lifted you into an old-fashioned bathtub on legs with a slanting back, which gave a supportive back and headrest.

The patient was washed and rinsed, lifted out onto the stretcher, dried on the stretcher, covered with a sheet, whisked back to the room, rolled off the stretcher into bed, and then an attendant took over from there. Not every bathroom had a bathtub. Some were just lavatories, and each lavatory was fitted with parallel bars for assistance.

Before I knew it, Thanksgiving Day had arrived, and I was disappointed that Harry could not come down for the holiday. It would have been quite an expensive trip, though, so I contented myself with looking forward to having Harry bring Kris down for Christmas. Several National Foundation executives were present for the Thanksgiving banquet. President Roosevelt's favorite accordionist, Graham Jackson, came up from Atlanta for the program, and after dinner, he came into some of the rooms to entertain patients who were unable to attend the banquet. Unfortunately, I did not have enough time up to go to the dining room, but Thanksgiving dinner served in the rooms was just as pleasing to the appetite, I am sure, for it was a wonderful dinner.

Everyone at the Foundation received phone calls from home eventually, and that was always an exciting event. East Wing 2 had a phone that could be used for making outgoing calls, and there was one in each office on each floor. If you happened to be in bed when your phone call came through and needed a lot of assistance like I did to get out of bed, your bed and all was pushed out into the hall and you received your call in the hall, right in bed.

There was never much privacy about anyone's long distance phone calls. Everyone did so much talking about their families at home anyway that after a long distance call, friends always gathered in your room to hear all the news about each member of your family.

Among the patients in residence while I was at the Foundation, was a young girl from China. She had been a patient for a year and was getting ready to go to New York for a short course in radio work before returning to China. Before she left, her folks called her from China. Everyone on the floor had been alerted for Kathy's call that evening, but it did not come in until 11:00 P.M. and everyone was in bed. However, everyone with open doors and within hearing distance was all agog over the strange conversation.

Harry and Kris were making plans to spend the Christmas holiday with me. I had been given permission to spend a long weekend with them at the Warm Springs Hotel, so I arranged to rent a portable wheelchair from a girl who had two of them. Reservations at the hotel had to be made well in advance, for there were many visitors for the holidays and the hotel was none too large. Polio patients were frequently guests at the hotel, and a ramped entrance was just one of the many conveniences for the patients.

Harry and Kris came down by train and arrived early in the afternoon two days before Christmas. Harry looked a little weary and white, and I found out later that he had due cause for looking a bit frayed around the edges. It seems that Kris has been terribly train sick the night before, and neither of them had had much sleep. It was Harry's first attempt to travel alone with our daughter. They made out pretty well, though—much better than I would have anticipated under the circumstances.

I was ready to leave when my family arrived, and Harry watched the orderly lift me into the chair to refresh his memory of how it was done. Prior to my treatment at Warm Springs,

Walking Isn't Everything

Harry had always had assistance in carrying me, so he did have something to learn. By this time, I was used to being bounced around by just one orderly, so it was a comparatively easy job. We called for one of the local taxis to come and get us. Taxis are in great demand in Warm Springs, and the drivers are always happy to lift you in and out of the cab if need be. In fact, they know a great deal about handling and assisting polios.

It was my first trip out of the Foundation in an upright position where I could see things, and I felt quite happy going over to the hotel. Kris was a little quiet, for her, but mostly because she was a tired girl.

When we got over to the hotel, we re-trimmed a small white artificial tree that Harry had sent to me two weeks previous for our room at the Foundation, and which we brought to the hotel to bring the Christmas season closer to us. We had an early dinner, and we turned out all the lights except those on the Christmas tree, so that Kris could get to sleep early. It was good to be with my family again, even though we were not at home.

I had mastered my arm slings pretty well by Christmas time, so my progress was very noticeable, but I did have one difficulty during our holiday. I still was not used to the low back on the portable wheelchair, and when I used the arm slings, I again had that old feeling of falling backwards. It was not as bad as it had been at the wedding, for I knew I was strung up with arm slings and could not possibly fall out, but it made me a little uncomfortable and awkward. When I got back to the Foundation, it was time to order my own wheelchair. I was glad of the Christmas experience in a portable wheelchair, because it enabled Lynn and me to know that I needed the added support of an extension back on my own chair.

I was successful in interesting Harry in a shopping trip in a nearby town on the day before Christmas. We set out complete with arm slings and lapboard, and though it was not an odd sight at all down there, it was something that would stop traffic elsewhere. I think the most fun of all was going shopping in the dime store, because it had been over two years since I had been in one. I do not think there is a woman alive who does not like to go into a dime store and poke around.

We really needed a horn, for Harry had the wheelchair to pilot and an eye to keep on Kris. The town was crowded with patients from the Foundation with their families, but we could not stay out too long because I still was not able to sit up for any great length of time. It was impossible to be put in a wheelchair without getting a few wrinkles in my slacks, and after I had sat on the wrinkles for a while, they made pressure points that would start to pain. My endurance was improving right along, but it was far from what I desired at Christmastime.

Walking Isn't Everything

CHAPTER **16**

Progress is Beginning to Show

We shared Christmas dinner at the hotel with friends from the Foundation. Harry had brought some of Kris' presents along and I had picked up a few at the Foundation gift shop, so her Christmas was quite complete and very exciting for her. After we talked with my mother long distance, our day was complete.

The holidays passed so quickly that before we knew it, it was time for me to return to the Foundation and for my family to return home. It took a few days for most of the patients to get back to normal. Charlotte had been fortunate enough to be able to go to her home, which was in Florida and not too far away, so we had lots to talk about after the holidays. That kept us from being too nostalgic and lonesome for our homes and families.

Shortly after Christmas, my own wheelchair, which Harry's folks had bought for me as a Christmas present, arrived. It was fitted with special attachments to accommodate my own particular involvements. It was an Everest-Jennings chair, which was the standard make usually ordered by the Foundation for its patients. It was upholstered in red leather, the chrome sides of the chair were removable, and it had brakes. It was fitted with overhead arm slings at the brace shop, and they added the extension back and put hooks on one side of the back so that the back of the chair could be opened and folded back. The chair back was fashioned in this manner to make one more way for me to get into the chair.

After my own wheelchair arrived, Lynn started to work on practical things, so to speak—a semi-remedial type of therapy. She tried to find the easiest way for me to be as functional as possible in my own home.

We tried washbasins for height and ways that I could wash at one. We tried a wheelchair geared to just one wheel for hand movement, thinking that I might be able to wheel my own chair with my best arm. My left hand and arm were of no use whatever in wheeling, and we learned that my right arm was not strong enough to enable me to make much headway. The chairs that could be wheeled with one arm necessitated a lot more arm strength in the first place. We decided it would be a long time, if ever, before I could use a chair of this type, but it was gratifying to have had the opportunity to try one. Now, I am able to wheel my chair enough to turn myself around, so perhaps I have the needed strength to make progress with the one-arm gear now. However, our home is small, and with our present domestic schedule, I have not felt an urgent need to attempt the change.

From January until I went home, about three afternoons a week were spent in preparing me for home life where I would be dependent upon my housekeeper alone many times for assistance. Lynn ordered a sliding board from the brace shop, for it is a real friend to a great many polios. It is a board about one-half inch thick, approximately twelve inches wide, and thirty inches long. Both ends are beveled, and the board is varnished and then highly waxed for slickness.

There are several ways to use sliding boards, and some patients are able to use them themselves to get from a wheelchair into bed, or vice versa, and in assisting them in getting in and out of a car. In my case, the wheelchair is wheeled up alongside the bed, which we made sure was about the same height as the wheelchair. The side of the chair next to the bed is removed, and one end of the sliding board is slid under my wheelchair cushion as far under my hip as it will go, and the other end of the board rests on the bed. Whoever is putting me to bed stands in front of me with their knee between my knees, with the chair footrests raised to enable the person to get a good firm footing. I put my arms around their neck and they slide my hips from the cushion by means of the board onto the bed, and half of me is in bed. The board is then removed, and my feet and legs are swung into bed. Lynn was a small girl, and she did not have bit of trouble getting me into bed by this method.

Our big trouble, we found, was in getting me out of bed. We tried to reverse the process by which I got into bed, but I did not seem to have enough muscles to hold myself well enough to make it an especially safe procedure. The outcome of our trials was the decision to take the chair to the brace shop and have the back made to open. This made a sure-fire method of getting me into the chair available, and while it is not a difficult procedure, it does take a little time to do it.

The wheelchair is backed up to the side of the bed, braked, and the back opened up. Then one end of the sliding board is slid under the wheelchair cushion and the other end rests on the bed, thus bridging the gap between the seat of the chair and the bed. Then I am slid around until I am lying crosswise in bed. This is where the time element enters into it, because with one person doing it, my shoulders are moved, then my hips, and then my legs. Of course, each portion of my body can only be moved a little at a time. None of it is hard work; it just takes time.

When my body is in a straight line, my legs are lifted over into the chair and I am lined up straight with the wheelchair. I am then pulled by my ankles down into the proper position in the chair, and the back is raised so that I am in a sitting position. Once I am in a sitting position, I can hold myself up away from the back of the chair while the board is removed and the back hooked up.

Since Harry is usually at home when I get up and his method of putting me into the chair is to pick me up and toss me into it, we seldom use the sliding board method. However, it is a necessity as a precautionary measure.

We also practiced getting me in and out of the lounge chairs at Georgia Hall. However, I must say that since I have had my own wheelchair, I have never had the slightest inclination to sit in a lounge chair, when I am visiting or at home. I was put in a lounge chair in our living room once to try out a new foam rubber cushion we had put in it. Although it is a very comfortable chair, for my needs it just is not equal to my wheelchair. For this reason, whenever we go out and the wheelchair does not happen to be with us, I stay in the car.

Before a patient was dismissed from Warm Springs, his functional ability was tested and graded. I remember a few things the test included, such as tying a package, threading a needle, and dialing a telephone. In general, most of the professional effort at Warm Springs was directed toward making the patient as self-sufficient and as functional as possible, and if you have any particular problems in your home, they are always glad to help you with them. There are plans available for a wheelchair house, which we brought home with us and have longingly viewed, but we have never been in a position to do anything about building it.

Lynn asked permission in January to use hydrotherapy in addition to treatment that I was already getting and got an okay from Dr. Bennett. We felt that it was quite a successful way of treating my arms. I enjoyed every minute of these pool treatments after my usual apprehension of anything new.

Everyone took a bathing suit to Warm Springs as part of his or her equipment, and mine was a pre-polio cotton strapless creation. I am sure that my atrophied body did not do justice to the bathing suit. Charlotte was successful in sewing some ties together to make a strap to tie around my neck, but we had quite a struggle with it. We found that she was fixing it about once a week to keep it together, but we were determined that it was going to last through my hydrotherapy, because there was no doubt in my mind that I would ever be a bathing beauty again.

You meet people from all walks of life at Warm Springs. While I was there, among the patients numbered a couple of doctors' wives, a restaurant owner, a professor from Yale University, a dentist, several lawyers, a missionary who was in India when she got polio, and I have already mentioned the girl from China. There were many boys and girls of school age, both high school and college, so the campus was always buzzing with romances.

There are also a great number of common ordinary homemakers such as myself. A common utterance around Warm Springs is that polio affects only brilliant people. This observance has all the earmarks of being a rumor started by a polio.

Fast friendships often formed among the patients. They all had one thing in common— polio. One of the ways ex-patients of Warm Springs could keep in touch with one another was through the Eaters Club, which a group of patients started a few years ago.

When one becomes a member of the Eaters Club, he automatically extends his hospitality by offering a meal to any member of the club who happens to call you while passing through your hometown. I remember reading in the Wheel-Chair

Review, the paper published by the patients at the Foundation, that one patient called on a friend expecting a free meal but did not find his friend at home. Before he left, he wrote a note deriding his friend for not being at home and implying that he left deliberately so he would not have to buy a meal. The would-be host, after reading the note, wrapped up a hamburger and sent it to his friend by return mail.

We still see quite a few of our friends that we met at Warm Springs, and I still correspond with a few that I do not see.

I was getting stronger constantly, and by the end of February, Lynn felt that we had gone about as far as we could. I went to clinic, eagerly anticipating my dismissal. Charlotte had been released a few days before and she was leaving at the end of the week. That heightened my anxiety to be on my way home, too. Dr. Britt was holding clinic that day, and when Lynn told him she thought we had gone as far as we could, he nodded his head and took up my progress reports to recheck.

When the doctor looked up and said that he thought Miss Denecke would be able to go home as soon as her husband came down and learned her treatment, I immediately burst into tears and tried to say thank you. Lynn started to whisk me out, but the doctor stopped us long enough to ask me if I was crying because I did not want to leave, and I assured him that it was just because I was so happy. It was really a joyous day for me, for in spite of my admiration for the Foundation, there is still no place like home.

I had been hinting for several weeks to Harry that I thought I would be dismissed some time in March, so it was not any real surprise to him, but I just could not wait to call him. I remember that I was very disappointed when he said he could not leave the next day. In fact, I thought it took him a long time to get there, when in reality, it was probably not more than four days.

Harry brought his movie camera with him, and he took movies of Lynn administering my therapy treatments. My hand exercises in particular were quite intricate, and he wanted to be sure that he had an accurate record. He was able to record on film the greater share of my treatment, which was a big help to him after we got home. We were there about three days while he was learning my treatment.

I was able to eat in the dining room those three days while Harry was there, which was quite a treat for me. This was possible because all my treatment schedules had ceased, so my time up for meals did not interfere with anything.

I said my goodbyes the night before I was scheduled to leave the Foundation, and it was then that one of the push boys paid me a valued compliment. When I thanked him for his helpfulness, he said, "Why you can't go home—you haven't been to the walking court yet." He was amazed when I told him I was one of the ones who were not going to walk again. The push boy's compliment was very nice, I thought, and it made me feel that at least I knew I did not look different from any of the others who were more fortunate in their involvement.

Walking Isn't Everything

CHAPTER 17

Home Once Again

We left early in the morning to start for home by train, and the Warm Springs ambulance drove us to Atlanta. When we arrived at the station, we went down the freight elevator to the tracks. We were told that the train was almost an hour late, so we wheeled back to the freight elevator, went up to the main floor, and everyone had coffee. When the train was finally due, we went back down the elevator to the tracks and Clyde, who was the ambulance driver from Warm Springs, picked me up from the cot and carried me into the bedroom on the train. We were all set to go home.

The trip was most enjoyable. I was able to sit on the backrest and see out the windows, and it was almost like traveling before polio again. At least, I had the illusion that it was. We left Atlanta in the middle of one morning, and we arrived at home about 8:00 the next morning.

Harry had arranged to have the same ambulance that had transported me on my previous rides meet us. They were on hand with plenty of blankets, for there was quite a change in temperature from what we had left in Georgia. That particular morning was very blustery and snowy.

Once again, my family was all bouncing up and down when the ambulance stretcher was carried in, but how good it seemed this time to be picked up from the stretcher and put into my wheelchair, rather than being plunked into bed.

My folks were there, and breakfast was waiting. My mother had been injured in a fall right after I left for Warm Springs and had not been very well since, so she had not been able to visit me while I was gone. Consequently, I had my wheelchair and arm slings to show off.

I remember how pleased I was to be able to drink my coffee that morning from a cup, instead of having to use a glass and straw. We have since found that a plastic cup is easier than pottery or china for me to handle, because the material is lighter. Also, plastic cups are usually simply designed, which means that they often have a square, large handle opening that makes for a surer grip.

The trip had not tired me at all, so after breakfast, Mother helped me arrange Kris' belongings back in her room, which had been vacated by Miss Rene. Kris also had quite a number of Christmas gifts to show me that I had not seen.

That year, I never did get Christmas gifts straight in my mind due to all the confusion and I imagine several people remained un-thanked for their kindness to us. It was wonderful to be home again, and I was anxious to get into some things that I could not possibly have seen to in pre-Warm Springs days. My father had contacted Fanny Mae for us, and she was coming the next day, so Miss Rene left that morning to go to another job.

I know many of my casual acquaintances were disappointed at the outcome of my treatment at Warm Springs, for frequently they would ask on their first visit or call after my return, "Do you walk now?" When my answer was "no," there was usually a letdown tone discernible. It is hard to explain to someone who is not familiar with my capabilities just what Warm Springs did for me, and is still doing, for that matter.

When you are as dependent upon someone for as many things as I am, walking ceases to be as important to you as it is to other people. The use I regained of my hands and arms was gratifying beyond telling. Physical comfort in normal breathing and the mobility that had been achieved by the use of the wheelchair more than made up for my inability to walk again. When almost everything has been taken away by polio, everything, every little thing, that is restored to you is like a miraculous blessing, for you never forget how it was in the beginning of polio paralysis. As handicapped as I am, others at Warm Springs were worse, so I realized the full worth of each little improvement.

The next day, Fanny Mae came as arranged. Harry got me up, and Fanny Mae and I decided that she could get me back into bed on the sliding board, so he went on to his office. Fanny Mae was a person who was very proud of her work, and I believe she really enjoyed taking care of me. She was also very determined. She used the sliding board and got me into bed just beautifully. I do not know whether I was surprised or not—I guess I just expected that she would. She said it was no effort at all, and we were both very pleased with ourselves.

I explained to Fanny Mae the method by which I was able to get into the wheelchair, so that afternoon she asked me if I would like her to get me up. I thought it would be a pleasant surprise for Harry to find me sitting up, so I let her get me into the chair.

I have always thought that if I had been fortunate enough to have had a great deal of money, I could not have possibly wished for a more devoted or willing person to care for me personally than Fanny Mae. However, there was housekeeping and cooking to do also, and as the weeks went on, we began to have difficulty. Our main trouble arose with the cooking.

Fanny Mae just was not used to being supervised with her cooking, and since I was now able to be up and looking around, I found that I was getting back to wanting things prepared the way our family particularly liked them. It was lots of fun for me to be able to help a little bit, but unfortunately, Fanny Mae seemed to resent my intrusion in her kitchen.

Maybe I was too anxious to exercise my newfound abilities, but as the weeks progressed, I found that Fanny Mae's resentment upset me a great deal and that it depressed me. She had a funny habit of shrugging her shoulders like one will do when one is about to give up. She would not be told anything—it had to be her way or not at all. Ultimately, I thought it was best to let her go.

There were many days following Fanny Mae's dismissal that we were sorry about it, because we had a long series of help problems after that.

CHAPTER 18

Help Problems—We Had Them

We had one young girl who was with me a day before I noticed that she had a skin condition on her hands. I asked her what the trouble was, and she said that she did not know. I told her that I would appreciate it if she would see a doctor about it, since she had to handle me and I would be uncomfortable if the condition were contagious and I contracted it. That evening, she went to her doctor, and afterwards she called me and told me that using strong soap and bleach caused the condition.

The doctor had suggested that she keep her hands out of water for two or three weeks, and she asked if I would hold the job open for her. I told her I was afraid that could not be done, but I suggested that she ask the doctor if she could work with rubber gloves. She called me back and said that she could wear rubber gloves, provided she wore white cotton ones underneath.

The next day, she came to work with her two pairs of gloves, and everything was fine. However, the second day came along, and when I noticed she had not cleaned the bathroom, I made some comment. She informed me that she could not do it that day, because she had not brought her gloves. She had not had time to wash out her cotton gloves the night before, so she did not bring them, and she was not going to put her hands in any water. It was beyond any stretch of my imagination to be able to figure out how she thought she could take care of our house and me that day without getting her hands in water. We finally got it straight that the work had to be done, gloves or no gloves, but I am certain things got a "kitty-wash" that day.

I remember one other trick this same girl pulled while she was with us. After the dishes were washed one evening, I was sure I heard her walking into the utility room and dumping the dishwater in the laundry tub. I was puzzled at this unusual procedure, so I called to her to come back to the bedroom so I could verify what I had heard.

She said, "Oh, yes, I emptied it in the laundry tub because I had already washed the sink." I asked her then if she had scoured the laundry tub. She looked amazed and said, "No."

I explained to her that just because the laundry tubs were not white and shiny was no reason to assume that they magically dispelled grease and that if someone happened to want to wash out something after she had gone, they would be surprised with a greasy mess.

I could tell by looking at her that she thought I was just too funny. She had told me that one of her previous jobs had been in New York City in an apartment hotel, where she had been hired to keep some woman's collection of "what-nots" dusted and her personal laundry done.

I am afraid I did not quite come up to this young woman's idea of a languishing invalid, or she to my idea of a housekeeper, so we parted company with one more domestic.

The most unusual experience I ever had with help has never ceased to amaze me. I had called my mother on the telephone and I was having a nice, long conversation with her, when I heard a rumbling noise coming from what I thought must be the kitchen. I asked Mother to hold the line while I called Cindy to ask what the noise was. I called a couple of times and got no response, and all of a sudden, it dawned on me that the noise I had been hearing must be Cindy snoring, but loudly.

It struck me as rather funny at first, so I laughingly told my mother about what had happened. However, she was not the least bit amused. She said I had better try to call her again and get her awake. After calling at least a half-dozen times, as loudly as I could, I still did not have Cindy awake.

I gave up finally and told Mother that she had better try to call my neighbor on the telephone to have her come in and wake Cindy, because the telephone was not in the correct position for me to be able to hang it up and dial it to make another call. However, we had one difficulty in that arrangement. I had called Mother, and the connection could not be broken until I hung up the telephone.

Mother had to go to her neighbor's house to use a telephone to call my neighbor. When my neighbor came in, she and I had a good chuckle about it, for she had walked right past Cindy, who was sleeping at the kitchen table with her head in her arms and had not awakened even when the door opened. My neighbor was apprehensive about how she should go about awakening Cindy, because she thought she might wake up frightened and swing at her or something.

We finally decided that she should walk past Cindy and give the kitchen door a loud bang, and then go home, looking through the kitchen window before she departed to see if the noise took its effect. The bang of the door did have the desired effect, but when I told Cindy of the bother we had to go to because she had gone to sleep, she was not the least bit concerned. In fact, a couple of days later she went to sleep again.

I learned my lesson from the first incident, and I made sure that the phone was now within my reach at all times.

This time when I heard her snoring, I was able to dial the operator and ask her to call my neighbor once again. Cindy's attitude was still insolent regarding her habit of going off to sleep, so Harry and I decided that she was not reliable enough to leave me with, so that was the end of her stay with us.

Whenever I hired help, I always tried to make it clear that we wanted someone who planned to work a while, because it was pretty hard on me to teach someone how to take care of me and then have them leave in a few weeks. However, my efforts along that line seemed to be wasted.

One girl whom I foolishly hired gave me a full page of references that I could have checked. However, her appearance was quite pleasing, she was a healthy-looking girl, and about the age that I had in mind, so I hired her without checking the references.

I think she had been with us two or three weeks when I heard her openly calling about another job. When she told me she was leaving, she explained that she liked her job all right, but that she wanted to go on to something else. She said she liked to learn a little bit about everything, and that she never stayed in a job more than two or three weeks. She felt that she had learned sufficiently about her various jobs in that length of time, and now she was ready to move on from this one to something else. This made me think back to the page of references that she had offered me, and I learned from that experience to always check at least one reference.

We had some amusement with the cooking. One morning, one of our neighbors brought over a small basket of freshly picked cherries, and since cherry pie is a favorite with Harry, I told our current help, we would have cherry pie for dinner that evening.

We went over the pie recipe together, and I asked her if she had the cherries all ready for the pie, and she said that she had. I thought at the time that she had not had much time to do much with them, but I let it go. When we had dinner that evening, my father was eating with us, and I asked him how the pie was. He said it tasted very good, but he found some pits in it. I looked startled, and decided I had better take a bite myself. Sure enough, the cherries had not been pitted. Daisy said she had never made fresh cherry pie before, and it had never occurred to her that there were pits in the cherries.

We have had some sorry cooks. I think the poorest excuse for a cook we had was an older woman whom I hired in desperation, at the same time thinking that at her age, she should at least know how to cook. She had not done much housekeeping for other people, but she needed the job badly.

I found, much to my amazement, that she had never made Jell-O. It became apparent very shortly, also, that she had never opened a can of baked beans, either. The baked beans that she served us were in the form of soup—apparently, she had added a can of water to them as you would to a can of condensed soup.

She was the one who set herself a place at our table, which, to begin with, was only halfway set. Harry and I were so surprised to find that she had set herself a place at the table that Harry found himself getting up and down to complete the table setting while she sat and shoveled food into her mouth.

The next night, Harry decided it would be easier for him to cook, so he told her she could go home. I found it was quite a task to explain tactfully to her that, although we were not what are commonly known as snooty people, it just worked out a lot better if she were available to wait on the table. As I remember, she did not last very long anyway, but she certainly did afford us some startling moments while she was with us.

We had another girl who was recommended to me because, although she was young and had not done any housekeeping for other people, her mother had been in a wheelchair for several years and the care of the mother had fallen mostly upon this nineteen-year-old girl. I thought that this time I would be able to dispense with a lot of the usual explanation concerning my personal care. However, the first time she put me on the bedpan, I found that I was quite uncomfortable and I could not quite figure out what she had done wrong. The next time I used the bedpan, I noticed that she had put the pan on the bed backwards. I asked her if that was the way she had handled the pan the time before, and when she said yes I knew why I had been so uncomfortable the first time. She had put the pan under me hind side forward.

I just did not have the nerve to ask her if that was the way she had been panning her poor mother all those years. In the days that followed, I tried to instill in her mind some of the easier ways of doing things that I had learned through the years of my illness so that she could apply them in her own home in the care of her mother. I know I was never successful.

Finally, we did find an excellent girl who was what we wanted in every way, except that she never could learn to put me back to bed. I think that her trouble was that she was afraid she was going to hurt me. It was not that she was not strong or healthy for she could work like a demon. She had a pleasing disposition and was interested enough in our daughter to be good with her. She would see that Kris minded, but at the same time, make Kris want to mind her. Perhaps that was because she had a little boy of her own.

After Myrtle had been with us a couple of months, she found that she could not find anyone to take care of her son any longer, so she had to leave. However, I could always rely upon Myrtle to come back and help when we were having a change of help, which she still does to this day. We were quite disappointed when we found that Myrtle was leaving, and after that, we had a couple more girls come and go.

Walking Isn't Everything

CHAPTER 19

Della

My mother would always try to come out and help us on the days when we were between help, but Mother had not been well since her fall while I was at Warm Springs. She had been having terrific head pains all summer, and in September, she had a severe attack that acted similar to a stroke with intense pain. She finally consented to go into the hospital for examination and possible surgery. When life looks the darkest, hope usually seems to step in, for I will always remember that Della came to work for us the day before Mother's surgery. She has been with us since, and her dependable presence helped carry me through the long months of Mother's last illness when I felt so frustrated by my inadequacy.

Della was very anxious to find a job, and when she was told at the agency that I was in a wheelchair, she expected to find a little old woman. Consequently, she was quite surprised when she arrived for her interview to find a young woman parked in a wheelchair. I asked her if she could start right away, and she said she would be glad to.

When Della prepared our dinner the first night, it was unbelievable to me to have things go as smoothly as they did.

Harry and I agreed that if the first day was any indication of her ability, we surely hoped she would stay.

We were more and more pleased as the days went by. Everything went along very smoothly. Della was able to get me into bed without any trouble, Kris because extremely fond of her, and she seemed to fit into our household beautifully. Some people are resentful of suggestions and directions from someone who is not working right along with them, no matter how kindly the suggestions are offered. I found this to be true with some of the help I had had, but from the very beginning, I was never aware of that difficulty with Della. She told me that she was raised in a fashion similar to the situation at our house, for her mother had ten children and weighed well over two hundred pounds, so the mother accomplished much of the work in their home by sitting and directing the children. She also remembers her father telling that she might as well do things the way her mother was telling her to do them, explaining that her mother was sitting and looking at just the work to be done, so that it was easier for her to see the best way to do it.

I think it might be interesting to most people to know how our housekeeping is managed. Now, I get up about eight hours a day—four hours in the morning and four hours in the evening, with the afternoon spent resting in bed.

Harry usually gets me into the chair after Della has breakfast started, and while he finishes getting dressed, Della helps me finish my dressing. Harry and Kris usually breakfast together, and when Kris is off to school, Della and I have our coffee. That is the time I usually plan the day's work. I always want to get some things done while I am up, for I am still keenly interested in my family and my home. If I can help, I do; if not, I supervise. I still know the answer to where things can be found when one of the family asks.

When we clean closets and drawers, Della takes things out of them and the articles that need inspection are put on my lapboard so that I can go over them. I have trained myself to keep complete track of Kris' wardrobe—what is in the laundry, what is waiting to be ironed, and what is clean in the drawers. Kris tells me when a button comes off or something tears, and I in turn remind Della on one of our sewing mornings.

Neither Della nor I is experienced at sewing. Our mothers both spoiled us in that respect. Last winter we did manage to make Kris a more-than-passable Indian costume for a school play. We cut our own pattern, and between us, we did the sewing by hand.

I try, about once every week or two, to go over the refrigerator and kitchen cupboards with Della in much the same way we do drawers and closets. Della always jots down articles that need replacing in the kitchen, for I make out the grocery list and Harry does the shopping. Sometimes, we foul up and think we have something on hand, only to discover that we are out of it when we are ready to use it. I am sure that happens in the best-managed households, and our borrowing trips to neighbors are no more frequent than anyone else's are.

Della likes to cook and like myself, enjoys trying new recipes. We take a lot of ribbing from the family when we serve some of our concoctions. We do a fair amount of baking, and if the mixer can be used, Della measures the ingredients while I hand-turn our almost worn-out mixer which cannot turn itself anymore.

Silver polishing is usually my job exclusively, for I manage it quite well. Keeping Kris' shoes polished is another thing I usually do myself. Harry takes the laundry to a launderette for washing once a week on his way to the office. We sort it at home, so all he has to do is put it in the machines. It is dried and folded there and ready for him to pick up on his way home. Things are usually folded so neatly that we have long since given up ironing everything but the essentials.

Walking Isn't Everything

Della used to iron in my bedroom and we would watch television while she was doing it, but it seemed that we would no sooner get clothes spread out all over the room and someone would come to visit me. Then we would have quite a scramble straightening up. We have moved since I came home from Warm Springs, and since then, the ironing board is always set up in the basement.

I try to devote at least a half-hour to complexion care each morning. I find it very necessary because of my inactivity. I can always work on this while helping Della verbally. I try to get back to bed before noon so that I am settled when Kris comes home for lunch and I am free to listen to her chatter. Very often, we all eat lunch in the bedroom. I cannot do much in bed, except read pocket-sized books or watch TV, so that is the way I usually spend my afternoons. My friends all know I am free then, so the phone frequently keeps me busy, too. Della goes on with the usual routine tasks and dinner preparation. Harry gets me up for dinner when he comes home, and with Kris helping Della with the dishes, she is usually ready to leave about 6:45 P.M.

Our household runs very smoothly, and a lot of my peace of mind is due to Della's just being Della. I have tried the same method of supervising with other help, and it is just impossible to use a flexible routine with most of them. A lot of our success, I know, stems from a genuine liking for each other. I sincerely wish that every handicapped person could be as fortunate as I have been in finding so capable a person to be his or her legs and arms.

CHAPTER 20

Things I Have Learned in Five Years

I think we spend our evenings as thousands of other families spend theirs. We frequently go for rides, play games with Kris, have company, or each of us is busy doing something of his or her own liking.

As the years accumulated, one by one, we learned the easiest, the best, or the quickest way, as the occasion warranted, to live with polio. One thing we did away with was the old footboard that was the length of the bed. Harry saw the small ones that were used at Warm Springs as footboards on stretchers. He decided that there was no need for the long footboard we had been using, because it had always let in a lot of draft on his side of the bed, as naturally he did not sleep with his feet flat against it as I did. We found that by using a small one, approximately one foot wide, it was quite suitable and eliminated a lot of the draft from his side of the bed.

Another of my problems has to do with shoes. Like all women, I became tired of the Girl Scout oxfords that I had purchased at Warm Springs. I rather fancied a different style shoe—perhaps a moccasin type oxford in color, which would be appropriate for wear with slacks. I had a great deal of difficulty in getting my foot into a shoe that did not unlace. I happened to notice in one of the magazines a very attractive moccasin type oxford in a suede-like finish. It came in many colors and had a sponge rubber insole. I was quite interested, so I ordered a pair. This turned out to be a very satisfactory investment and since then, I have worn nothing but these shoes. They are not expensive, so I am able to have two or three colors for variety in my wardrobe.

My mother had sent me a couple of nylon sweaters while I was at Warm Springs, and they worked out very well for me. Anyone who has had much experience with washing wool sweaters knows that it is very easy to ruin them, and with the various changes in help that I had, my nylon sweaters have weathered the storm beautifully.

My wardrobe now consists mainly of nylon sweaters, tee shorts, and slacks. Mother took in a couple of my blouses on the shoulders and I have hemmed them to wear on the outside of my slacks. It is difficult to keep blouses tucked in when I am lifted and carried. I find maternity jackets work out very well too. They have a flattering fullness and they are made to wear on the outside.

We developed a new hair-washing system. Harry bought a tray similar to those used in the beauty shops, and we found that by backing the wheelchair up to the kitchen sink and having someone hold the tray up to my neck, we could attach a spray to the sink faucet and shampoo my hair very easily and quickly. One morning a week is devoted to my hair, and that is all the attention it needs.

I have always enjoyed talking on the telephone, and that was a pleasure I had been looking forward to when I came home from the hospital the first time. We had an extension phone installed in the bedroom so I could talk either in bed or in the iron lung in the living room. This worked out fine until we built the porch, and since I frequently spent the day there, I missed the telephone. We consulted with the telephone company and they suggested the jack and plus system. We had three jacks installed with just one telephone instrument that could be plugged into any of the three jacks, wherever I might be. We are all pleased with our telephone system, for it affords privacy as well as convenience. Upon further investigation, we learned that an ivory instrument was appreciably lighter in weight, thus easier for me to handle.

Last winter was our first winter to use an electric blanket, and I cannot praise it enough. My circulation is naturally poor, and sometimes in the winter, my feet and legs would be cold all day long and it was always hard to get to sleep at night with such cold feet. If I used a hot water bottle to warm my feet, it eventually became heavy as well as cold and would waken me. The last straw was when I found myself so heavily laden with covers to keep warm, that I could not move my arms up and down during the night. Harry did not want all the covers on him that I had on me, so we always had trouble keeping what belonged to me on just my side.

Finally, last October, Harry brought home this wonderful electric blanket with double controls for my birthday. It has completely solved all of our warmth problems. We now only need one blanket. Harry's side can be turned as low as he prefers, while mine is turned as high as I need it for comfort. It also eliminates having a supply of various weight covers available for seasonal changes. I feel it is one of the most satisfying expenditures we have ever made.

I have continued with occupational therapy since I have returned from Warm Springs. Some of the handcraft was very interesting for Kris. Harry bought her a thirty-inch stool, which is an excellent height for her to sit alongside my wheelchair and work on the lapboard with me. She gets a big kick out of stenciling, and she was interested when I suggested that she stencil pillowcases for her bed—something she could use.

We made many potholders, which Kris insisted upon taking around the neighborhood and selling. We usually work on our handcraft after dinner, and it often turns into a family affair.

I have progressed to the point where I can sew a moderate amount, also. It is quite easy for me to hem anything if I use a rather coarse needle. When I first started to sew, my needle had to be stuck into a block of plywood to hold it still for me to thread. I no longer need to bother with that, since some of my polio shakes seem to have left me.

The fact that my hands do not shake so much helps to make my handwriting more legible and very similar to what it used to be. My only trouble is that I usually tire long before my thoughts are all down on paper. If I am writing a letter and do not put it away until another day when I become tired, it is not at all hard for the reader to detect the exact point at which I did tire.

No mention of letter writing would be complete without my telling of my very good friend, Betty Isom, who has helped to make this book possible. We had been friends for several years before I got polio, but after I got polio, Betty more than proved the real meaning of friendship. There were very few weeks that she missed visiting when I was in the hospital, and it was not long before all of the girls in iron lungs knew Betty, too. Visitors can be important to you when you are hospitalized for a long period.

After I came home from the hospital, Betty continued to come out, and she was always looking for something to do to help Harry as well as myself. We have tried to make it a rule never to burden our friends with any of our polio problems.

However, when someone so obviously wants to help, we are more than appreciative.

Some time after my first few months at home, the thought suddenly occurred to me that, since Betty had been a secretary before her marriage, why could I not dictate my letters to her? I mentioned it to her and she was more than pleased to be able to do something specific, so for over two years, my friends heard from me through Betty.

When I decided that folks might be interested in our polio story, I asked Betty if she would be interested in taking the story in shorthand and typing it. As we got into it, we found that two heads are better than one, and it has been one more task we have enjoyed doing together.

Walking Isn't Everything

CHAPTER **21**

Kris

Kris was able to join the Brownies the fall after I came home from Warm Springs. After I talked with our neighborhood chairperson and she told me how hard it was to get mothers to cooperate, I offered to do any telephoning that the troop might have to be done, in order to do my part in scouting. This was an enjoyable job for me, because it gave me an opportunity to become acquainted with the other mothers and to get a more accurate idea of what the troop was doing. It enabled me to be a little closer to Kris, and it helped her to know that, in spite of polio, her mother was helping out, too.

I am very often complimented because Kris is such a healthy, active nine-year-old and shows no obvious scars from having her mother in a wheelchair. I must return a great share of the compliment to Kris. She minds me very well, and it is seldom that she takes advantage of my obvious inability to use physical strength to punish her or to keep up with her activities. We have had our episodes, however, and one in particular I will always remember.

I had been home from the hospital for several months, and one day, Kris and I happened to be at home alone until

155

Walking Isn't Everything

Harry came home from work. I hated to keep Kris in to stay with me, working on the theory that my polio must never seem to spoil things for her. I told her she could play outside but to come in every now and then to see me.

The last time she came in, I told her it would soon be dark, so not to go away. It did get very dark soon, and Kris did not come in. I listened for her voice and could not hear it anywhere. By this time, the house was pitch black, I was petrified wondering where she could be, and the phone was not within my reach.

I spent a miserable half-hour until Harry came home, and as he set out to find Kris, she came out of the house next door. She said the shades were drawn at the neighbor's house, and she did not know it had become dark. Kris had been told not to go into neighbors' houses without asking. I had explained to her that we did not have time to chase around finding her, and when we looked, we wanted to be able to see her. We checked her closely for a few days after that, and I soon found that I did not have to worry about Kris forgetting again.

Kris accepts my being in a wheelchair very matter-of-factly, and so far, she shows no self-consciousness around her friends when they are here or when we go to school. She brings her problems to me without hesitation, for I impressed upon her from the beginning that what I could not do, I could always see that someone else did do. She also has an excellent relationship with her father, which she will learn to appreciate more as she grows older. From the time I came home from the hospital, I have worked very hard to teach Kris to be as independent as possible. I have always felt that the more she could learn to do for herself, the better off she would be.

Both Harry and I try to be very careful to see that our daughter has a well-rounded life. Our friends are more than helpful, too. For instance, now, Kris's Brownie leader and her family take Kris to Sunday school with them each week. Kris enjoys belonging to their family for that part of the day.

My own church work again consists mostly of telephone work. I have always been profusely thanked for any of my efforts to any organization, when in reality, I feel I should be doing the thanking for being able to enjoy the outside contacts that these efforts afford me.

Walking Isn't Everything

CHAPTER 22

Life Goes On

Mother was acutely ill for most of the winter of 1950–1951. She seemed to be progressing for a few months after her surgery, but gradually she lost footing and was very ill for about six months. This was a very difficult time for us all. More than once, I have been glad that this happened after I had been to Warm Springs. Now I had the wheelchair and was able to visit my mother when she was in the hospital, and later at home. In addition to Mother's illness, Kris and I had had the flu, and though it was not serious with me, it lasted a long time.

The strain of the difficulties we had encountered that winter was beginning to tell on all of us, and we decided in the spring that we would undertake to visit Marguerite and Bob Myers. We asked Harry's folks to take Kris for us, and we set out to drive about 185 miles to the Myers' home, complete with all our paraphernalia.

Surprisingly enough, I stood the trip very well. We used small pillows under my hips as we had used when I first came home from the hospital. All I required was a little boost off the pillows about every hour or so. When I was getting my boost,

Harry moved my legs either up or down to give them a change of position, and we managed quite well.

We stayed about ten days, so I had plenty of time to rest in between trips there and back. Marguerite lives upstairs, and our greatest problem was getting me up the winding, steep stairway. Once I got up there, I stayed until I was ready to go home. The trip did us all much good, because while we were there, Harry was able to get away for a few days to take care of some business matters that had been pending. It was good to see old friends again, and we truly enjoyed ourselves.

When we got home, we found my mother much worse. The remaining three months that my mother was with us were difficult ones for me to sit more or less idly through, but by then I knew that Mother's death was inevitable and it was something we all had to accept. I did not want Kris to be unduly upset, and that thought helped to steady me.

More than a year has passed now, and as the completion of this summary of my experiences with polio neared, I began to look around for something else to do that would be interesting— preferably a simple business within the scope of my limited capabilities.

One day I saw a woman being interviewed on television who ran a successful babysitters registry. The idea intrigued me enough that I inquired extensively into the business and its possibilities. The more I learned the more interested I became, and that is how my Rock-A-Bye Sitters Registry was born.

The registry has been operating for several months now, and it has been very well received within our city. I enjoy it; I am able to handle it with a minimum of help from my husband and Della; and I am showing a profit already. There is every indication that I will have an enjoyable and lucrative business from my venture.

160

I feel fine, my friends and mirror tell me that I look just like I did B.P. (before polio), so I hope that I have been able to give encouragement to other polio victims who think that life might not be worth living. Both Harry and I feel that we have a very full and rich life, in spite of the restrictions that severe polio has brought to us.

Walking Isn't Everything

Appendix A

Graphs on the Occurrence of Polio in the United States

1954 Annual Statistical Review

National Foundation for Infantile Paralysis

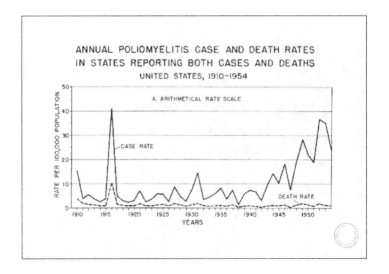

ANNUAL POLIOMYELITIS CASE AND DEATH RATES
IN STATES REPORTING BOTH CASES AND DEATHS
UNITED STATES, 1910-1954

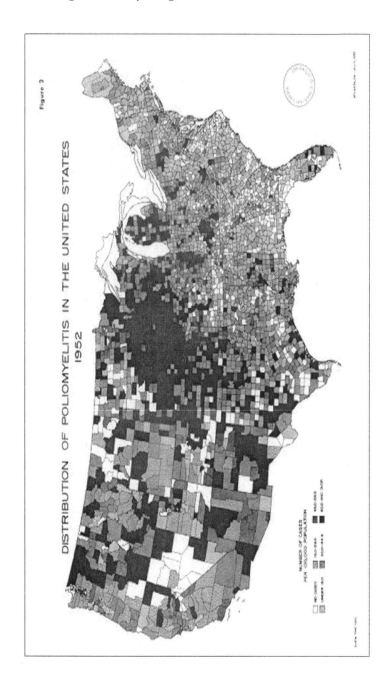

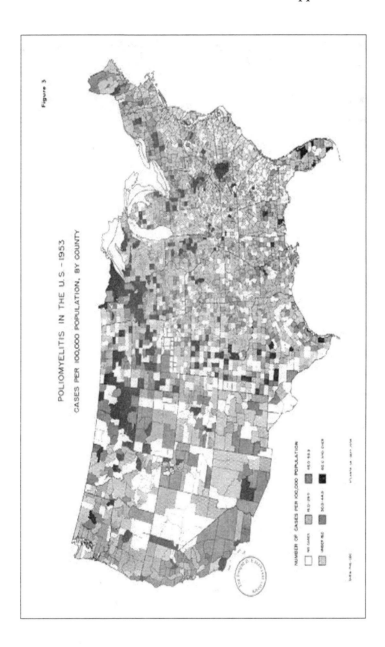

POLIOMYELITIS IN THE U. S. – 1953
CASES PER 100,000 POPULATION, BY COUNTY

Figure 3

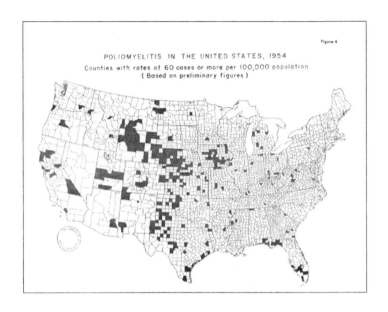

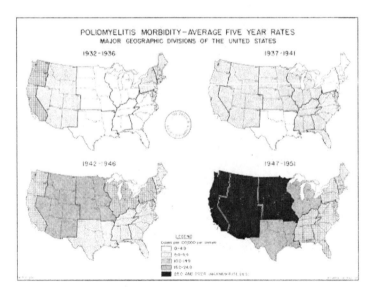

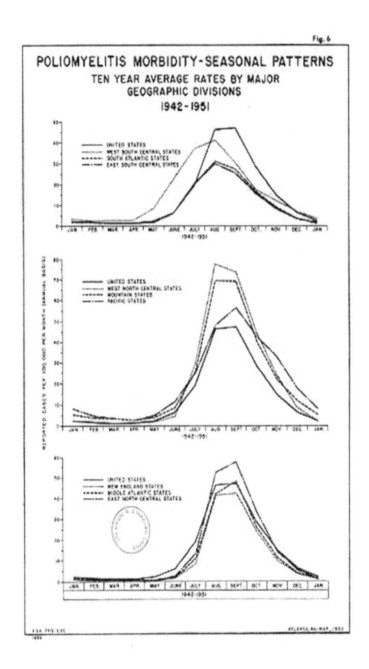

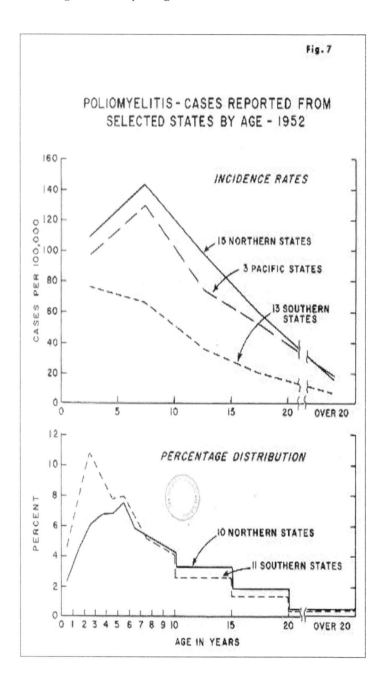

Fig. 7

POLIOMYELITIS - CASES REPORTED FROM
SELECTED STATES BY AGE - 1952

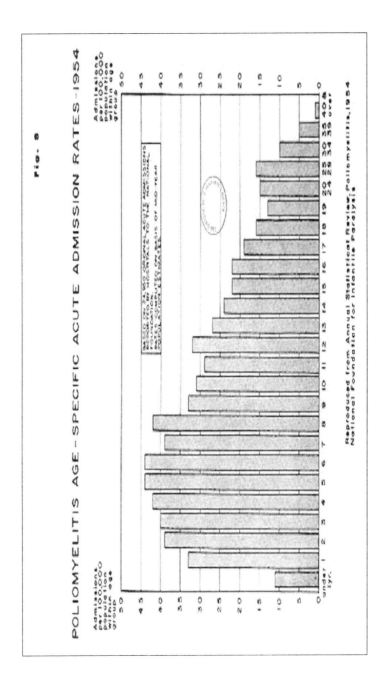

Fig. 8

POLIOMYELITIS AGE-SPECIFIC ACUTE ADMISSION RATES-1954

Reproduced from Annual Statistical Review, Poliomyelitis, 1954
National Foundation for Infantile Paralysis

Walking Isn't Everything

Appendix B

1947 Twentieth Anniversary Annual Report, Georgia Warm Springs Foundation

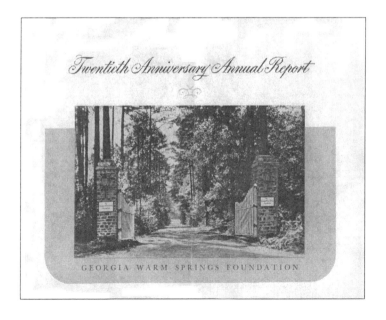

171

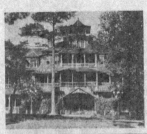

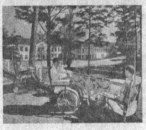

Foreword

TWENTY YEARS ago, on July 28, 1927, the Georgia Warm Springs Foundation was incorporated as a non-profit institution for the treatment of the after-effects of infantile paralysis.

It was frankly an experiment. Nobody knew at that time how much could be done to ameliorate the crippling caused by poliomyelitis, to devise treatment that would enable those who were handicapped to lead full and useful lives. One man believed these things were worth finding out that Warm Springs was the place in which to plant the seed of the idea.

From the dream of Franklin D. Roosevelt has emerged the first and largest complete medical unit dedicated exclusively to treatment of infantile paralysis. Its origin, its growth through two decades, the part played by the American people in its progress and far-reaching effectiveness are told in this Twentieth Anniversary Annual Report.

Because today the Foundation has reached the milestone of twenty-one years, it is fitting to review the history of the years between 1927 and 1947, as well as the record of the twentieth year of its existence. One can trace in these pages the forward steps of the institution founded by the late President, its significance as a symbol of the nation's fight against infantile paralysis.

Many things have changed in twenty years. The Foundation's creator is no longer its most affectionate and popular guest. But both the Georgia Warm Springs Foundation and the National Foundation for Infantile Paralysis, founded eleven years later, are living memorials to Franklin D. Roosevelt that have won the affection and support of 140,000,000 people. Gleaming backward through the years one sees the pattern of a growing crusade to stamp out infantile paralysis, a crusade which will continue until there is no more.

Basil O'Connor
President

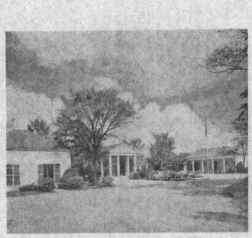

Center in the Georgia Warm Springs Foundation, showing Georgia Hall, built by contributions from citizens of Georgia.

[2]

The Twentieth Year

As the Georgia Warm Springs Foundation marked its twentieth birthday in 1947, it was giving service to more men, women and children who had infantile paralysis than in any of its previous years. A total of 799 persons, almost 100 more than were admitted in 1946, was cared for at Warm Springs.

Progress was made in other ways: expanded professional education, new facilities such as an enlarged kitchen in Georgia Hall, a national clinical conference of medical authorities held on the Foundation campus. But the most fitting sign of growth was in the roster of patients from forty-three states of the United States, the District of Columbia, Puerto Rico and fourteen foreign countries. The average daily number in residence throughout the year was 152, twenty-four more, each day, than during the preceding year. They received 55,706 hospital days' care.

The larger number was made possible by ex-

pansion of facilities completed late in 1946 providing eighty-six more beds and enlarged space for other purposes.

Most of those who were treated during the twentieth year received financial assistance, as in other years. Of the 799 there were 547 patients, receiving 40,575 hospital days' care, who fell in the category of Aid Patients. Most of these were helped by their local Chapters of the National Foundation for Infantile Paralysis, supported by the March of Dimes. It is the Chapters' job to provide the means for adequate medical care and treatment for all those who cannot meet the full cost of infantile paralysis without financial aid.

At Warm Springs no distinctions are made in care or housing between Pay and Aid Patients. Their particular financial classification, as a matter of fact, is known only to the personnel of the Foundation in charge of financial arrangements. There are no patients from whom any

[3]

profit is derived, since maximum rates do not exceed cost of care for the individual patient.

More patients applied for admittance to the Foundation than could be accepted, despite increased facilities. Those admitted were selected on the basis of their need for the special facilities provided at Warm Springs, with due attention given to the availability of similar facilities near the patients' homes.

In general, those unable to obtain similar care in or close to the communities where their families live and those whose physical involvements present opportunity for study and improvement of treatment techniques are selected.

All patients are admitted upon application to the Registrar, with a complete medical case history from the attending physician accompanying each application.

For a detailed record of patients during the twentieth year, see the tables on Pages 26 to 28.

PROFESSIONAL TRAINING

Georgia Warm Springs Foundation is a training center for professional workers in the field of treatment of the after-effects of infantile paralysis. To it each year come physicians, nurses, physical and occupational therapists, social workers and others seeking to observe modern methods of treatment.

The Physical Therapy Post-Graduate School, which is part of the Foundation, is one of the most important in the nation. During the twelve months ended Sept. 30, 1947, a total of thirty-six qualified physical therapists, graduates of approved schools throughout the country, participated in three-month intensive courses in polio care. Three such courses were given, starting on the first Mondays of January, April and October. Following each course, selected students were asked to remain an additional three months.

Post-graduate physical therapy students receive sixty dollars a month and full maintenance while training, through a grant from the National Foundation for Infantile Paralysis for this purpose.

The course is designed to train qualified phys-

[4]

ical therapists in special phases of polio care such as muscle strength evaluation, body mechanics, muscle re-education, use of active and supportive apparatus and walking re-education. When they leave Warm Springs, these physical therapists are able to spread their new knowledge of treatment in all parts of the country.

In addition, 26 physicians, nurses, social workers and other professional personnel took short courses in polio care during the year.

SPECIAL EVENTS

The Little White House, where Franklin D. Roosevelt lived when he visited Warm Springs while President of the United States and in which he died in 1945, was turned over to the State of Georgia on June 25, 1947 by the Foundation, to whom Mr. Roosevelt had willed it.

Ceremonies marking the occasion were held on that day, attended by statesmen and officials from Atlanta, Washington and many states of the union, as well as distinguished representatives of foreign countries.

Thus the Little White House and adjacent land became the property of the people of the State of Georgia, to be developed as a national and international shrine. The Franklin D. Roosevelt Warm Springs Memorial Commission, composed of prominent citizens of the state, was allotted funds from the Georgia Legislature to develop the site.

Work was begun during the summer of 1947 to prepare the house and grounds for visitors the following year. Foundations and floors were being strengthened, the grounds landscaped for public use. An approach to the Little White House eliminating the use of Foundation roads by tourists is to be built. The furnishings and simple decorations of the house will remain the same as in President Roosevelt's lifetime.

A clinical conference for physicians interested in infantile paralysis was held at Warm Springs on Sept. 15, 16 and 17, 1947, to celebrate the twentieth anniversary of the Foundation with a

[5]

174

review of progress in the treatment of the disease between 1927 and 1947.

Visiting medical men from all parts of the country witnessed demonstrations of treatment given at the Foundation. Papers were read by medical authorities outlining the various phases of modern polio treatment.

The patients themselves staged the entertainment for visiting physicians, a musical presentation entitled: "The Wheelchair Revue."

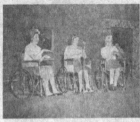

Three patients who starred in "The Wheelchair Revue."

[6]

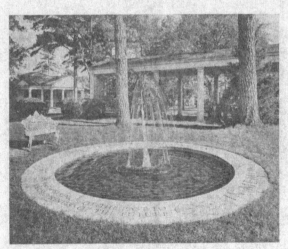

[7]

Walking Isn't Everything

The Story of Warm Springs

1927–1947

In the beginning there were the springs, gushing warm out of the earth in a silent sea of pines. There, legend has it, Indians of the Creek confederacy in Georgia, Alabama and northern Florida brought their wounded warriors—to bathe in the springs, after all other efforts to heal their injuries had failed. A stricken warrior was granted safe conduct through territories of hostile tribes, if his destination was "the warm springs." Thus, the springs became an influence for peace, a sort of inter-tribal sanctum in the Georgia wilderness.

The atmosphere of peace still pervades the clearing in the pine woods, known today throughout the world as the Georgia Warm Springs Foundation. In a sense, those who come there also are granted safe conduct through the suddenly hostile territory of the "normal" world to which they once belonged, from which they have become separated by their affliction by infantile paralysis. Their safe conduct pass is the

[8]

wish of their fellowmen to see them become well and strong again, a wish given reality through streams of dimes and dollars to ease the way.

Although any magical properties of the warm springs long have been discredited, the waters are used to a greater extent and for more wounded warriors than ever the Creek Indians could have imagined. They have become one of many routes to health and strength offered at the Georgia Warm Springs Foundation.

Geologists have explained how the rain that falls on Pine Mountain, several miles away, descends 3800 feet to a vast pocket of rock, is warmed by the inner earth and returned to the surface, at a rate of 800 gallons each minute and a temperature of 88 degrees F. Engineers have calculated it would require twenty tons of coal every twenty-four hours to duplicate nature's water-heating performance at Warm Springs. Thus it is that this spot naturally attracted, first, people who sought warm-water bathing for rec-

reation, later, cripples seeking warm-water treatment for their ills.

But it took another kind of magic to transform the Indians' warm springs and the white man's holiday retreat into the first and largest

hospital for the treatment of the after-effects of infantile paralysis, mother of the infantile paralysis movement in the United States.

It was the magic of a vision powered by one man, who dreamed it into being

HALF A CENTURY AGO...

. . . Warm Springs, Georgia, was a small summer resort for people seeking relief from sultry cities and air adulterated with smoke from multiplying chimneys of the new industrial age. There, on the site of a post tavern on a military highway leading to Columbus, Georgia, the Meriwether Inn did a thriving seasonal business. A large, rambling building with gingerbread on its roof line, gables galore, outlines in woodwork to shame an old-fashioned penman and contours unclassifiable in architecture, it welcomed two generations of guests who, in the early days, arrived by stagecoach from the railroad depot at Durand, Georgia. The nearest village was Bullochville, which took the name of Warm Springs in 1924.

In the early 1900's the automobile proved that it could take Georgians farther away for relaxation, and Meriwether Inn went into decline. By 1924 it had become a run-down resort,

still gracious with hospitality, still loved by a few who had known it in more fashionable days, but hardly to be suspected of future growth or national importance.

To Meriwether Inn, in the fall of 1924, came a private citizen from Hyde Park, New York. He was a man in the prime of life who had been stricken by infantile paralysis. His legs were useless. Improvement had been agonizingly slow for three years. But Franklin D. Roosevelt came to Warm Springs to try to overcome his crippling condition and to give the sleepy little village and the waning resort a new and meaningful destiny in the doing.

He didn't know that, then. Nobody knew. He came because his friend, George Foster Peabody, who had purchased an interest in old Meriwether Inn from its original owners, Charles Davis and his niece, Miss Georgia M. Wilkins, told him about a young man who had had infan-

[9]

176

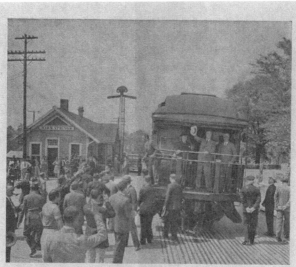

[10]   *Familiar sight in the 1930's; the President arriving at Warm Springs.*

tile paralysis, who swam in the warm springs and appeared to improve. Private Citizen Roosevelt stayed only a few weeks, but it was the first of many visits, visits which were to change not only his own life but the lives of many others who, like him, had had infantile paralysis. And here twenty-one years later fate ordained that his life's work should end.

THE IDEA WAS BORN...

. . . as Mr. Roosevelt swam in the public pool, located about 500 yards from the shabby elegance of Meriwether Inn. He was startled into belief in his own progress by the greater ease with which he was able to move his lame legs under water. He was discovering, for himself, the value of hydrotherapy, an ancient healing art, that today has become part of the flowering profession of physical medicine.

Not a scientist, and without medical background, Mr. Roosevelt could not explain *what* was happening, as he progressed after many patient hours of exercise in the warm, buoyant waters of the resort pool. He consulted the local country doctor, Dr. James Johnson; together they tried to figure it out on the basis of physical facts. Which muscles were used? How could one test their returning strength? The two men didn't find the answers — but they set the stage for later scientific work along these very lines.

Dr. Johnson, now consulting physician to the Foundation and still practicing in the neighboring town of Manchester, remembers a crude muscle chart prepared by Mr. Roosevelt that was used to guide other infantile paralysis victims as they came to Warm Springs to follow Mr. Roosevelt's example. For they came. How they came! By ones and twos, then five; finally, that first year, a total of seventeen patients — uninvited, unprovided for, drawn by accounts in the newspapers of Franklin D. Roosevelt's efforts to "swim his way to health."

One of the first of these was young Fred Botts of Elizabethville, Pa., a recent college graduate who had been studying singing in New York when infantile paralysis cut short his career. Mr. Botts, today Registrar of the Georgia Warm Springs Foundation, remembers vividly the bewilderment, the confusion, the misunderstandings of those old days. Regular resort guests protested the use of the pool by polio patients for fear of "catching" the disease, forcing Tom

[11]

177

Loyless, manager of Meriwether Inn, to bar even the use of the regular dining room to the "paralitic." These men and women seeking strength for their crippled bodies ate their meals for some time in a separate dining room in the basement of the Inn.

Mr. Roosevelt, on his own, built a small treatment pool twenty-five or thirty yards from the public pool where he and his "gang" could continue their unsupervised, unregulated, groping efforts to reduce their afflictions in the warm water of the springs.

But that wasn't enough, and Mr. Roosevelt knew it. He sought scientific appraisal of what was happening.

In 1926, having observed that other patients, too, thought they had been benefited by their sojourns at Warm Springs, Mr. Roosevelt invited Dr. LeRoy W. Hubbard, orthopedic surgeon of the New York State Health Department, to come down and take a professional look. Dr. Hubbard observed twenty-three patients for periods of from five to seven weeks each between June and December of 1926. At the close of the season, a detailed report of each case was sent to three

[12]

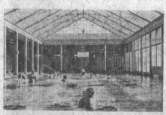

The glass-enclosed pool built in 1928, in use until 1952.

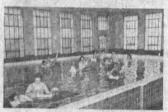

The present campus pool where all hydrotherapy now is given.

prominent orthopedic surgeons, all of whom had sent patients to Warm Springs. Each patient had seemed to improve, and some showed marked improvement.

That convinced the man from Hyde Park. His dream of a center Inn after care of infantile paralysis at Warm Springs had been growing;

now professional opinion gave sinews to the dream. With four other men whose interest he obtained, he formed the Georgia Warm Springs Foundation, a non-stock, non-profit institution. The incorporators were Mr. Roosevelt, George Foster Peabody, Basil O'Connor, Herbert N. Straus, and Louis McH. Howe.

THE NEW FOUNDATION . . .

. . . had two objectives:

1. To use the natural facilities of Warm Springs and the skill of an able, carefully-selected professional staff for the direct aid of patients.

2. To pass on to the medical profession and to hospitals throughout the land any useful observations or special methods of proved merit resulting from this specialized work, which might be applied elsewhere.

So it was, in 1927, that gentlemen in plus-fours collected their golf clubs and checked out of Meriwether Inn. Ramps replaced the front porch stairs, and men, women and children in wheelchairs, on crutches or with canes, checked in. Women in crisp white uniforms replaced women in sports clothes.

And an unseen guest checked into the old Inn, not as a transient but as a permanent resident. Her name was Hope.

IN 1927 . . .

Georgia Warm Springs Foundation consisted of the old Meriwether Inn, several guest cottages and the old resort pool. It was called "the Colony," because of its residential appearance. According to Reinette Lovewell Donnelly, one of the early patients, it "looked like any old-time hostelry in any quiet mountain resort of the Eastern states. Porch chairs, a great dining room,

[13]

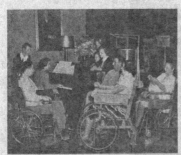

After-dinner music, home-grown variety, in Georgia Hall.

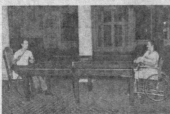

Ping Pong is a popular pastime at the Foundation.

[14]

with negro waiters, parked automobiles with state licenses from far and near, big trees of oak and pine, and under them a midget golf course. Only after a first look did you see the fleet of wheelchairs filled, for the most part, with youth, and the crutches, canes, braces. But nothing there seemed like a hospital or sanitorium. It had the spirit of a country club."

Nevertheless, in 1927, seventy-one patients were treated, and there was a staff of 110 medical and other Foundation employees.

Dr. Hubbard was the first medical director. He served until December 1, 1931, when Dr. Michael Hoke, Atlanta orthopedist, became Surgeon-in-Chief of the Foundation.

The Foundation grew rapidly, amazing the associates of the man from Hyde Park, who travelled frequently to Warm Springs with him, fired by his enthusiasm. Not even Basil O'Connor, to whom Mr. Roosevelt turned over the direction of Warm Springs in 1928 on becoming Governor of New York State, foresaw in those days what this Foundation was to be.

Mr. O'Connor shared his former law partner's expressed belief: "In my opinion it would be a mistake to think of the Foundation as just a hospital. It is all of that and more. . . ." But, in those days, before Mr. Roosevelt even had built his own cottage on the grounds and long before he had any intimation that he would occupy a Little White House there, who could have realized that the Indians' old healing springs and the run-down summer resort would be sponsored by the whole American people through a celebration of the President's Birthday each year, leading to the establishment of a public-supported National Foundation for Infantile Paralysis?

FIRST SIGNS OF GROWTH. . .

. . . were in 1928, when a glass-enclosed patients' pool was built with a gift from Mr. and Mrs. Edsel Ford. Then came the Norman Wilson Infirmary, a small building to house patients with incidental illnesses, built in 1930 at a cost of $10,000 raised directly by patients and their friends. It was named for a Philadelphia patient who had died shortly after he left Warm Springs. There followed, in 1933, Georgia Hall, the present administration building, built with $125,000 contributed by the citizens of Georgia, the state President Roosevelt regarded as his "second home."

Then, in 1935, came two dormitories housing forty-five patients. Kress Hall was built with funds largely donated by Samuel H., Rush H. and the late Claude W. Kress, and Builders' Hall with money donated by friends of the builders,

Hegeman and Harris of New York City. That same year a playhouse was created by remodel-

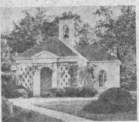

The Chapel at Warm Springs.

[15]

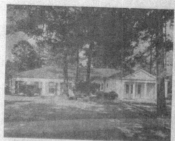

The school and occupational therapy building, built 1939.

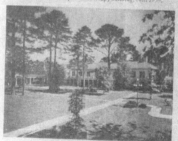

The Medical Building, complete orthopedic hospital.

ing the old outdoor dance pavilion of Meriwether Inn, through the generosity of the Hon. Frank C. Walker and the late Michael E. Comerford. It is here patients now see their movies every Monday, Thursday and Saturday, the films provided free of charge by Atlanta distributors. Here, too, the patients put on their own shows, hear visiting lecturers.

The Chapel was erected in 1937, the donation principally of Miss Georgia M. Wilkins, one of the former owners of Meriwether Inn and the springs.

The Brace Shop came into being in 1938. Here appliances are made according to doctor's prescriptions, fitted and adjusted to patients in residence. Hundreds of alumni come back every year for adjustment of their appliances, new braces, crutches and other aids to motion. The Brace Shop is famous, serving people throughout the nation. Its original size was doubled in 1946 and it is still growing.

The School and Occupational Therapy Building went up in 1939, gift of Mrs. S. Pinkney Tuck. Here are classrooms, library and a craft shop frequented by a large majority of the patients in residence.

Perhaps the biggest step forward was the opening in 1939 of the Medical Building, through which the Foundation became a complete orthopedic hospital. An average of 200 operations a year are performed in this building. Before 1939, patients requiring surgery had to travel to Atlanta, seventy-two miles away, for such services. On June 15, 1946, an east wing was added to the Medical Building, bringing the capacity of the building from 95 to 141. Thus a majority of the Foundation's patients has lived here since the middle of 1946.

Today's Physical Therapy Post-Graduate School was established in 1941. The next year the campus pool, where all hydrotherapy now is given, was erected with funds from an anonymous giver.

The old Meriwether Inn is no more. It was razed to make way for Kress and Builders' Halls. Some of the cottages still stand – one on the campus. There are thirty-six Foundation-owned cottages today.

The Foundation has become a complete community, a village unto itself. It comprises about 4200 acres of land, of which twenty-five are landscaped and tended, and includes what used

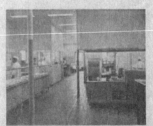

The Foundation's modern kitchen, finished in 1947.

to be the Roosevelt farm – 2500 acres, 100 of which are cultivated. There are ten miles of red clay road winding through this acreage, every mile of it maintained by the Foundation.

The Foundation has its own heating plant, laundry, commissary, fire department, even its own golf course and an 1800-volume library. Patients are transported from trains and airports by modern ambulance and passenger car.

[17]

TWENTY YEARS OF PROGRESS...

... have touched the clearing in the pine woods with a transforming finger. But it did not all happen at Warm Springs, Georgia.

The new buildings that went up, the new interest that mounted, the wider ripples of hope that spread from Warm Springs throughout the nation were made possible by the generosity of a people who shared the dream of the man from Hyde Park. For in 1932 they elected him thirty-first President of the United States, and in 1934 they became his partners in supporting the Georgia Warm Springs Foundation.

On January 30, 1934, the first Birthday Balls in celebration of the President's birthday were held throughout the land. They were sponsored by the American people for the benefit of the polio center then President had brought into being at Warm Springs. More than $1,000,000 was raised that first year – and it happened again in 1935, 1936, 1937.

By that time, the horizons of the dream had begun to grow.

The President continued to come to Warm Springs for periodic check-ups and treatment, living in the simple six-room house he had built on the grounds to 1932, the house destined to

be known as "the Little White House." His visits were among the happiest periods of his life. Each trip, from the moment he stepped down from the ramp from his special train at the tiny Warm Springs station, to be greeted by the villagers, until he drove himself in his blue automobile with specially-constructed driving controls, followed by Secret Service men, for a last look at Shiloh Valley from the top of Pine Mountain, he was "one of the Foundation gang" – that man from Hyde Park, seeking strength and health and happiness.

But much as he loved the place, he realized it was not the whole answer to the problems of infantile paralysis patients.

Obviously, the Foundation, with its limited number of beds, could not take care of all the infantile paralysis patients in the country. Were there enough other places equipped and staffed to give good treatment for the after-effects of infantile paralysis?

Then, too, new victims of the disease appeared each year. What were scientists doing in the field of research to find out what caused infantile paralysis and to discover a preventive or possible cure?

[18]

THE ANSWER...

... came on January 3, 1938, when the National Foundation for Infantile Paralysis was formed, with Basil O'Connor as president. The new Foundation, in the words of Mr. Roosevelt, was "to lead, direct and unify the fight" against infantile paralysis. Since that time, all the funds raised in January of each year have been for the National Foundation; the Georgia Warm Springs Foundation has been one of its grantees.

For some years a large percentage of Warm Springs patients, always preponderantly non-pay or part-pay patients, has been financed by their local Chapters of the National Foundation. There are more than 2,700 such Chapters in the country, whose chief function it is to give financial assistance to infantile paralysis patients whose families cannot pay all the high costs of adequate treatment.

Many more are financed by these Chapters for care and treatment at hospitals in all forty-eight states which have opened their doors to polio patients. Many hospitals now have polio wards staffed and equipped in part with funds from National Foundation Chapters. Physicians, nurses, physical therapists, medical social workers, health educators, medical record librarians and others have been trained with March of

Dimes money for expert care and treatment of infantile paralysis patients, wherever they might be. Warm Springs is not the only place where excellent modern treatment for infantile paralysis can be obtained today, although it still is the only complete hospital exclusively for the after-care of infantile paralysis cases.

Today, too, one of the largest medical research programs in history is under way, financed by the people of the United States through the National Foundation for Infantile

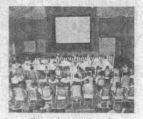

Manicures shown three times a week.

[19]

Paralysis. President Roosevelt had appointed a research commission in 1947 to ascertain the need for nationally coordinated and financed research seeking to solve the mystery of infantile paralysis. He tested his own idea that it was needed, much as he had tried out the idea of a treatment center at Warm Springs by getting professional advice. The recommendations of the commission have been followed with projects totalling almost $15,000,000 for research and education since 1938, results of which — in knowledge of

the disease and its proper care — have been noticeable everywhere, even though the ultimate goal of prevention or cure has not yet been attained.

All this activity, the improvement that has come about throughout the nation in twenty years, was touched off by the vision of the man from Hyde Park and the cooperation of the millions of citizens whose destiny he guided for almost thirteen years. Its birthplace was Warm Springs, Georgia.

THE SPIRIT OF WARM SPRINGS

Many changes have come to the Georgia Warm Springs Foundation since 1927, but in some ways it hasn't changed at all.

"It is not the policy of the trustees to develop Warm Springs into either a hospital or a sanatorium," reads an early report, "Warm Springs does and always will offer people the facilities to live normal lives – to receive treatment and to be instilled with new hope, a new philosophy of thinking and a mental therapy which, after all, is the heart and soul of physical therapy."

Of course, it is a hospital now, and an excellent one, but that spirit of normalcy still prevails within its walls and among its colonnades, none the less.

When the sun is bright on the clean white sides of Georgia Hall, and pine tree shadows fall across the green campus, stretchers appear on the balcony porches of the Medical Building; wheelchairs gather on the concrete walking area under the balcony; ambulatory patients find a place in the sun. Even then, you are struck with the resort-like, the college-like spirit of the place. For these are men and women, boys and girls, who have come to improve their physical condition and to grow, study, learn, play, make friends, fall in love, be happy while they are doing it.

They are following a high tradition. For each of them, the founder of Georgia Warm Springs

[20]

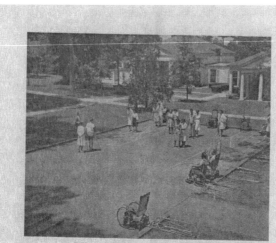

Walking area where patients learn to use their new muscular powers.

[21]

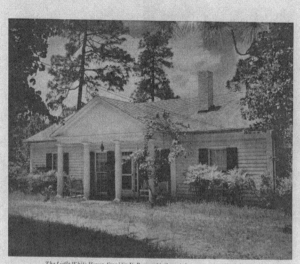

The Little White House, Franklin D. Roosevelt's Georgia home, now a national shrine.

[22]

is an inspiration. He, too, did what they are doing—his life, which was a great one, was bound up in this place. And he learned to rise above his afflictions. They feel they will, too.

To them the newly-won prominence of Warm Springs as an historic site is personal distinction. The white-shingled cottage caressed by thick foliage that has been empty since April 12, 1945, is more than a national or international shrine to them. It is the focal point of their interest, the visible evidence that Franklin D. Roosevelt once lived here.

The Little White House itself is a simple, though charming, building set at the side of a hill which is one of many surrounding the Foundation campus. Its unpretentiousness, the informality of its furnishings, the vista of woods and valley glimpsed from its stone terrace are typical of the man who built the house, lived in it, died there. But they are typical of Georgia Warm Springs Foundation, too. It's all of one piece.

Pine-panelled walls, big stone fireplace, hooked rugs, overflowing bookcases—these are everywhere at the Foundation. All the patients, and the Foundation staff as well, belong to it and it belongs to them.

They don't stay here long, most of the patients. The average stay is 190 days. For most, Warm Springs performs no miracles, nor do the patients expect miracles. They may walk out of the gates with or without braces, may leave knowing they are scheduled to return later on. But they carry with them that sense of belonging to a special fraternity, all the members of which understand a little better what they have done and what they must do.

Theirs is a proud faith in themselves to face the future with the spirit of Warm Springs, of the man in the Little White House.

[23]

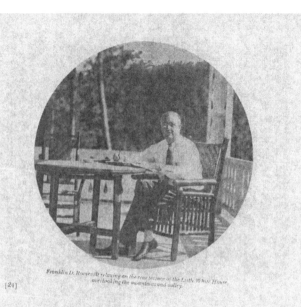

Franklin D. Roosevelt relaxing on the rear terrace of the Little White House, overlooking the mountains and valley.

[24]

Farewell

The day before Franklin D. Roosevelt went away from Warm Springs for the last time, he got in his familiar blue car and drove out to Dowdell's Knob, a flat shelf atop Pine Mountain which was his favorite look-out station. He dismissed his guests and companions, sat there alone behind the wheel of his car, looking over the green sweep of Shiloh Valley to the pinkish hills. He sat for two hours.

Nobody knows his thoughts that day, nor ever will. But those who knew him best at Warm Springs recalled something he had often said.

"You know," he used to say, "when we get hopeless patients, we ought to bring them out here and let them look at this valley. If they can do it and not be inspired, then we'll know they are really hopeless — not before."

A look at the Georgia Warm Springs Foundation, over the valley of its twenty years of existence, also presents a vista of hope.

[25]

184

Appendix B

Statistics of the Twentieth Year

I. GEOGRAPHICAL DISTRIBUTION OF PATIENTS

Alabama	40	Oregon	1
Arkansas	14	Pennsylvania	20
California	2	Rhode Island	1
Colorado	1	South Carolina	21
Connecticut	3	Tennessee	43
District of Columbia	2	Texas	58
Florida	61	Utah	8
Georgia	171	Vermont	1
Illinois	53	Virginia	20
Indiana	9	Washington	2
Iowa	4	West Virginia	18
Kansas	6	Wisconsin	1
Kentucky	7	Wyoming	1
Louisiana	8		
Maine	2		
Maryland	13	*Territorial and Foreign*	
Massachusetts	14	Canada	5
Michigan	3	China	2
Minnesota	20	Colombia	1
Mississippi	18	Cuba	7
Missouri	7	Denmark	1
Nebraska	1	Dominican Republic	1
Nevada	2	El Salvador	4
New Hampshire	17	France	2
New Jersey	32	Mexico	4
New Mexico	22	Nicaragua	2
New York	6	Puerto Rico	3
North Carolina	31	Peru	1
North Dakota	10	Turkey	1
Ohio		Venezuela	2
Oklahoma		Union of South Africa	1
			799

[26]

II. AGE AT DATE OF ATTACK

Less than age 1 year	27	Age 6 through 10 years	112
Age 1 year	43	Age 11 through 15 years	143
Age 2 years	32	Age 16 through 20 years	116
Age 3 years	31	Age 21 through 30 years	142
Age 4 years	37	Over 30 years	21
Age 5 years	45		**799**

III. DURATION OF PARALYSIS AT TIME OF ADMISSION

Less than 1 month	15
1 to 3 months	66
3 to 6 months	68
6 to 12 months	97
Over 1 year	553
	799

IV. AGE GROUPS OF PATIENTS IN RESIDENCE

1 through 4 years	38
5 through 9 years	92
10 through 14 years	144
15 through 19 years	189
20 through 24 years	140
25 through 29 years	96
30 through 39 years	72
Over 39 years	30
	799

[27]

185

V. APPLIANCES

Plaster Room:
Casts:
Extremities 495
Wedgings 463
Spicas 91
Jackets 81
1130

Corsets 376

Brace Shop:
Brace Shoe Attachments 2202
Brace Repair and Adjustments 1945
Miscellaneous 753
Inter-Department Jobs 495
Special Shoe Alterations 595

Everett Canes and Crutches (Pr.) 391
Overhead Slings 290
Long Leg Braces 259
Long Leg Splints 210
Opponens and Hand Splints 190
Wheelchair Repairs and Alterations . 154
Cork Raises 144
Miscellaneous Canes and Crutches (Pr.) . 128
Corset and Jacket Attachments 66
Short Leg Braces 63
Canadian Canes and Crutches (Pr.) ... 55
Spinal Jackets 44
Special Braces and Appliances 37
Wheelchairs 27
Blount Frames 12
7858

VI. X-RAYS MADE 1555

VII. OPERATIONS PERFORMED 279

VIII. PHYSICAL THERAPY DEPARTMENT

Supervised Walking and Steps 29,456
Exercise Treatments:
At Pools 10,025
At Infirmary and Medical Building .. 21,938   31,963
Radiant Heat Light 3,750
Massage 2,594

Paraffin Baths 1,150
Muscle Examinations 815
Thermo-mat 688
Ultra-Violet 369
Whirlpool 215
Diathermy 153

IX. LENGTH OF STAY

Average length of stay of patients present during the period (this includes
any uninterrupted visit which was begun prior to October 1946 but was
extended into the period) .... 86 Days
Uninterrupted longest length of stay .... 971 Days

[28]

HASKINS & SELLS
CERTIFIED PUBLIC ACCOUNTANTS

1 EAST 44TH STREET
NEW YORK 17

ACCOUNTANTS' CERTIFICATE

GEORGIA WARM SPRINGS FOUNDATION:

We have examined the balance sheet of Georgia Warm Springs Foundation as of September 30, 1947 and the related statements of revenue and
expenses and fund reserves for the year ended that date. Our examination was made in accordance with generally accepted auditing standards
and included such tests of the accounting records and such other auditing
procedures as we considered necessary in the circumstances.

In our opinion, the accompanying balance sheet and statements of
revenue and expenses and fund reserves present fairly the financial condition of the Foundation at September 30, 1947 and the results of its
operations for the year ended that date, in conformity with generally
accepted accounting principles applied on a basis consistent with that of
the preceding year.

HASKINS & SELLS

January 9, 1948

[29]

GEORGIA WARM SPRINGS FOUNDATION

Balance Sheet, September 30, 1947

ASSETS

CASH	$ 187,079.93
ACCOUNTS RECEIVABLE	56,883.54
SUPPLIES	89,184.21
DEFERRED CHARGES	15,550.01
PROPERTY (It is not the policy of the Foundation to make provision for depreciation of property)	1,810,292.78
TOTAL	$2,146,490.47

LIABILITIES

ACCOUNTS PAYABLE OR ACCRUED		$ 24,999.31
FUND RESERVES:		
Special	$ 200,564.11	
General	1,922,927.05	2,123,491.16
TOTAL		$2,146,490.47

[30]

GEORGIA WARM SPRINGS FOUNDATION

Statement of Revenue and Expenses
For the Year Ended September 30, 1947

REVENUE (exclusive of grants)
From patients ($592,588.81) and from other activities at Warm Springs, Georgia
From donations and bequests

EXPENSES:

EXCESS OF EXPENSES OVER REVENUE FOR THE YEAR

[31]

GEORGIA WARM SPRINGS FOUNDATION

Statement of Fund Reserves
For the Year Ended September 30, 1947

	Total	General Fund Reserve	Special Fund Reserve for Improvement and Extension of Facilities at Warm Springs
Balance, October 1, 1946	$2,421,050.94	$1,984,437.71	$467,413.23
Additions:			
Donations received in memory of Franklin D. Roosevelt	14,956.47		14,956.47
Restoration of reserve for extraordinary repairs and renewals (created in a prior year)	40,000.00	40,000.00	
Grant from the Federal Works Agency for construction of new medical building (final payment)	17,158.00	17,158.00	
Grants from The National Foundation for Infantile Paralysis, Inc.			
For general purposes (applicable to the year ended September 30, 1946)	145,000.00	145,000.00	
For educational purposes (applicable to the year ending December 31, 1947)	21,115.00	21,115.00	
For functional occupational therapy program (applicable to the year ending December 31, 1947)	11,266.00	11,266.00	
TOTAL	$2,671,246.41	$2,169,270.71	$501,969.70
Deductions:			
Excess of expense over revenue for the year ended September 30, 1947	$ 240,719.86	$ 240,719.86	
Expenditures for improvement of facilities at Warm Springs	301,405.59		$301,405.59
Refund of unused portion of prior year's grant for educational purposes	5,650.00	5,650.00	
TOTAL DEDUCTIONS	$ 547,749.25	$ 246,343.86	$301,405.59
Balance, September 30, 1947	$2,123,491.16	$1,922,927.05	$200,564.11

[32]

OFFICERS

BASIL O'CONNOR, *President and Treasurer*

GEORGE E. ALLEN, *Vice President*

KEITH L. MORGAN, *Vice President*

WILLIAM F. SNYDER, *Vice President and Secretary*

STEPHEN V. RYAN, JR., *Vice President and Assistant Secretary*

FRED BOTTS, *Assistant Secretary*

C. W. BUSSEY, *Assistant Treasurer*

L. D. CANNON, *Assistant Treasurer*

RAYMOND H. TAYLOR, *Assistant Treasurer*

EXECUTIVE COMMITTEE

JOHN S. BURKE, *Chairman*

VINCENT CULLEN
JOHN C. HEGEMAN
CLARENCE G. MICHALIS

JEREMIAH MILBANK
BASIL O'CONNOR
LOUIS H. PINK

WILLIAM F. SNYDER, *General Counsel*
RAYMOND H. TAYLOR, *Executive Secretary*

[33]

Appenidix B

189

Walking Isn't Everything

Appendix C

1955 White House Press Release Regarding Polio

IMMEDIATE RELEASE April 22, 1955

James C. Hagerty, Press Secretary to the President

- -

THE WHITE HOUSE

Following are the Citations given today by
The President to Dr. Jonas E. Salk and the
National Foundation for Infantile Paralysis

The Citation for Dr. Salk is as follows:

Because of a signal and historic contribution to human welfare by
Dr. Jonas E. Salk in his development of a vaccine to prevent
paralytic poliomyelitis, I, Dwight D. Eisenhower, President of
the United Stated, on behalf of the people of the United States,
present to him this citation for his extraordinary achievement.

The work of Dr. Salk in the highest tradition of selfless and
dedicated medical reasearch. He has provided a means for the
control of a dread disease. By helping scientists in other
countries with technical information; by offering to them the strains
of seed virus and professional aid so that the production of vaccine
can be started by them everywhere; by welcoming them to his
laboratory that they may gain a fuller knowledge, Dr. Salk is a
benefactor of mankind.

His achievement, a credit to our entire scientific community,
does honor to all the people of the United States.

The Citation for the National Foundation for Infantile Paralysis is as follows:

1. Dwight D. Eisenhower. President fo the United States, present
This speical citation to the National Foundation for Infantile
Paralysis for its unswerving devotion to the eradication of poliomyelitis.

The American people recognize a debt of gratitude to the Foundation
And to its founder, the late President Franklin D. Roosevelt, whose
Personal courage in overcoming the handicap of poliomlitis stands
As a symbol of the fight against this disease.

Without the support and encouragement of the Foundation, the work
of Dr. Jonas E. Salk and of many others who contributed to the
development of a preventive vaccine could not have gone forward so
rapidly. The Foundation displayed remarkable faith in sponsoring
and determination in fostering their valiant effor for the health of
all mankind

The generous voluntary support of the Foundation by the American
people has been dramatically justified. In their name, I am privileged
to make this award to the Narional Foundation for Infantile Paralysis.

######

IMMEDIATE RELEASE   April 22, 1955

James C. Hagerty, Press Secretary to the President

- -

THE WHITE HOUSE

Supplement to the Citations Presented
by the President to Dr. James E. Salk
and the National Foundation for Infantile
Paralysis

(After introduction of Dr. Salk by Miss Hobby and reading
Citation)

The President: Dr. Salk, before I hand you this Citation,
I should like to say to you that when I think of the countless
thousands of American parents and grandparents who are
hereafter to be spared the agonizing fears of the annual
epidemic of Poliiomyelitis. When I think of all the agony
that these people will be spared seeing their loved ones
suffering in bed, I must say to you I have no words in which
I know...all 164 million Americans, to say nothing at all
The people in the world that will profit from your discovery.

I am very, very happy to hand this to you.

(After introduction of Basil O'Connor by Secretary Hobby and
After the President read Citation)

The President: And there, of course, remains the great problem
of rapid production, distribution on the fairest possible basis,
and to that problem as Secretary Hobby has said, you and many
others are working and contributing to carry the thing forward
until there is no more poliomyelitis remaining in the United States.
And I thank you and all the Foundation of which you are
President.

######

Walking Isn't Everything

Appendix D

**1953 Newspaper Article on Jean
Denecke**

Heads Baby Sitter's Agency

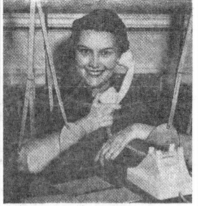

—Arella Studios

Mrs. Harry Denecke of 228 N. Lafayette, efficiently operates her Rock-a-Bye Baby Sitter's Registry from a specially equipped wheelchair which enables her to write and use the telephone. Stricken with polio six years ago, Mrs. Denecke inaugurated the agency in April of this year. It serves as an occupational therapy for the attractive business woman.

Parents Offered Answer to Baby Sitter Problem

By BETTY ZIMMERMAN
Women's Editor

Dearborn parents may not be aware that a valuable baby sitter's service available to them also serves as an occupational therapy for its founder and operator, Mrs. Harry Denecke, of 228 N. Lafayette.

Rock-a-Bye Sitter's Registry, organized in April of this year, is the answer to the timely issue that parents be assured of obtaining reliable sitters for their children.

It is also the answer to Mrs. Denecke's problem of keeping occupied to help her overcome the physical handicap of infantile paralysis.

Stricken with polio six years ago, Mrs. Denecke spent eight months in an iron lung at Herman Keifer Hospital and six months in the lung at home.

Following treatment at Warm Springs, Ga., the attractive woman returned to Dearborn to begin her period of rehabilitation.

One day while watching the "Welcome Travelers" show on television, Mrs. Denecke was particularly impressed with the story of a woman who overcame a physical handicap by organizing a baby sitter agency.

Thus, the idea for the Rock-a-Bye Registry formed in her mind. Mrs. Denecke instigated plans for her own such business which now boasts 52 registered clients and is licensed as

"However," Mrs. Denecke emphasized, "we have the personnel to handle at least twice as many clients."

Rock-a-Bye sitters are all capable adult women who are experienced in child care.

Mrs. Denecke personally interviews each sitter and checks their references.

"I am now making arrangements for each sitter to have a chest x-ray," she added.

Mrs. Denecke efficiently operates her agency from a specially built wheel chair with pulleys which enable her to use her arms and hands.

The energetic business woman also occupies her time by doing church work for Dearborn's First Methodist Church and by keeping a Girl Scout scrapbook for the area.

Mrs. Denecke lives in her attractive home with her husband, Harry, an employee of the United States Printing and Lithograph Company; her daughter, Kristin, 10, a student at Haigh School, and Mrs. Della Felmore, who has been her housekeeper and faithful companion for the past three years.

Bibliography of Works Related to Polio

[1] Aitken, Sally, Helen D'Orazio, and Stewart Valin, eds. 2004. *Walking fingers: The story of polio and those who lived with it.* Montreal: Vehicule Press.

[2] Alexander, Larry as told to Adam Barnett. 1954. *The iron cradle.* New York: Thomas Y. Crowell Company.

[3] Axtell, Agnes. 2004. *A polio memoir.* Martinsville, IN: Bookman.

[4] Banister, Betty. 1975. *Trapped: A polio victim's fight for life.* Saskatoon: Western Producer Prairie Books.

[5] Beisser, Arnold. 1990. *Flying without wings: Personal reflections on loss, disability, and healing.* New York: Bantam Books.

[6] ———1990. *A graceful passage: Notes on the freedom to live or die.* New York: Doubleday.

[7] ———1991. *The only gift.* New York: Doubleday.

[8] Berg, Roland H. 1946. *The challenge of polio: The crusade against infantile paralysis.* New York: Dial Press.

⁹ ———1948. *Polio and its problems*. Philadelphia, PA: J. B. Lippincott Company.

¹⁰ Black, Kathryn. 1996. *In the shadow of polio: A personal and social history*. Reading, MA: Addison-Wesley.

¹¹ Bruno, Richard L. 2002. *The polio paradox: Uncovering the hidden history of polio to understand and treat "post-polio syndrome" and chronic fatigue*. New York: Warner Books.

¹² Carter, Nancy Baldwin. 2002. *Snapshots: Polio survivors remember*. Omaha: NPSA Press.

¹³ Carter, Richard. 1966. *Breakthrough: The saga of Jonas Salk*. New York: Trident Press.

¹⁴ Cohn, Victor. 1975. *Sister Kenny: The woman who challenged the doctors*. Minneapolis: University of Minnesota Press.

¹⁵ Coughlan, Robert. 1954. *The coming victory over polio*. New York: Simon and Schuster.

¹⁶ Crawford, Dorothy H. 2000. *The invisible enemy: A natural history of viruses*. Oxford, NY: Oxford University Press.

¹⁷ Curson, Marjorie N. 1990. *Jonas Salk*. Englewood Cliffs, NJ: Silver Burdett.

¹⁸ Daniel, Thomas M. and Frederick C. Robbins. 1997. *Polio*. Rochester, NY: University of Rochester Press.

¹⁹ Davis, Fred. 1963/1991. *Passage through crisis: Polio victims and their families*. New Brunswick, NJ: Transaction Publishers.

²⁰ Fine, Michelle and Adrienne Asch, eds. 1988. *Women with disabilities: Essays in psychology, culture, and politics*. Philadelphia, PA: Temple University Press.

²¹ Finger, Anne. 2006. *Elegy for a disease: A personal and cultural history of polio*. New York: St. Martin's Press.

Bibliography of Works Related to Polio

[22] ———1990. *Past due: A story of disability, pregnancy, and birth.* Seattle, WA: Seal Press.

Fisher, P. J. 1967. *Polio story.* London: Heinemann Company.

[23] Fleischer, Doris Zames and Frieda Zames. 2001. *The disability rights movement: From charity to confrontation.* Philadelphia: Temple University Press.

[24] Fournier, Larry. 1988. *I did it! So can you!* Gilbert, AZ: Pussywillow.

[25] Freidel, Frank. 1956. *Franklin D. Roosevelt: The ordeal.* New York: Little, Brown and Company.

[26] Fries, Kenny, ed. 1997. *Staring back: The disability experience from the inside out.* New York: Plume.

[27] Galbally, Rhonda. 2004. *Just passions: The personal is political.* Nort Melbourne, Victoria: Pluto Press.

[28] Gallagher, Hugh G. 1998. *Blackbird fly away: Disabled in an able-bodied world.* Arlington, VA: Vandamere Press.

[29] ———1985. *FDR's splendid deception.* New York: Dodd, Mead, and Company.

[30] Gartner, A., and T. Joe, eds. 1987. *Images of the disabled, disabling images.* New York: Praeger.

[31] Goldberg, Richard Thayer. 1981. *The making of Franklin D. Roosevelt: Triumph over disability.* Cambridge, MA: Abt Books.

[32] Gould, Jean. 1960. *A good fight: The story of F.D.R.'s conquest of polio.* New York: Dodd, Mead and Company.

[33] Gould, Tony. 1995. *A summer plague: Polio and its survivors.* New Haven, CT: Yale University Press.

³⁴ Gritzer, Glenn and Arnold Arluke.1985. *The making of rehabilitation: A political economy of medical specialization, 1890–1980.* Berkeley, CA: The University of California Press.

³⁵ Hall, Robert F. 1990. *Through the storm: A polio story.* St. Cloud, MN: North Star Press.

³⁶ Halstead, Lauro S., and Naomi Naierman, ed. 1998. *Managing post polio: A guide to living well with post-polio syndrome.* Arlington, VA: ABI Professional Publications.

³⁷ Hawkins, Leonard C. 1956. *The man in the iron lung: The Frederick B. Snite, Jr. story.* Garden City, NY: Doubleday.

³⁸ Henrich, Edith and Leonard Kriegel, eds. 1961. *Experiments in survival.* New York: Association for the Aid of Crippled Children.

³⁹ Hillyer, Barb 1993. *Feminism and disability.* Norman, OK: University of Oklahoma Press.

⁴⁰ Huse, Robert C. 2002. *Getting there: Growing up with polio in the 30's.* Bloomington, IN: 1st Books Library.

⁴¹ Johnson, Mary. 2003. *Make them go away: Clint Eastwood, Christopher Reeve & the case against disability rights.* Louisville, KY: Advocado Press.

⁴² Kehret, Peg. 1996. *Small steps: The year I got polio.* Morton Grove, IL: Albert Whitman & Co.

⁴³ Keith, L., ed. 1994. *Mustn't grumble: Writings by disabled women.* London: The Women's Press.

⁴⁴ ———, ed. 1996. *What happened to you?: Writing by disabled women.* New York: The New Press.

⁴⁵ Kendall, Henry O. 1939. *Care during the recovery period in paralytic poliomyelitis.* Washington, DC: U. S. Govt. Printing Office.

[46] Kenny, Elizabeth 1955. *My battle and victory: History of the discovery of poliomyelitis as a systemic disease.* London, UK: Hale.

[47] ——1941. *The treatment of infantile paralysis in the acute stage.* Minneapolis, MN: Bruce Publishing Company.

[48] Kenny, Elizabeth, and M. Ostenso. 1943/1980. *And they shall walk: The life story of sister Elizabeth Kenny.* New York: Arno Press.

[49] Kingery, Kenneth. 1966. *As I live and breathe.* New York: Grosset & Dunlap.

[50] Kirkendall, Don and Mary Phraner Warren. 1973. *Bottom high to the crowd.* New York: Walker and Company.

[51] Klein, Aaron. E. 1972. *Trial by fury: The polio vaccine controversy.* New York: Scribner.

[52] Kluger, Jeffrey. 2004. *Splendid solution: Jonas Salk and the conquest of polio.* New York: Putnam.

[53] Kriegel, Leonards. 1991. *Falling into life: Essays.* San Francisco: North Point Press.

[54] ——1998. *Flying solo: Reimaging manhood, courage, and loss.* Boston: Beacon Press.

[55] ——1964. *The long walk home.* New York: Appleton-Century.

[56] Lake, Louise. 1971. *Each day a bonus: Twenty-five courageous years in a wheelchair.* Salt Lake City: Desert Book Company.

[57] LeComte, Edward. 1957. *The long road back: The story of my encounter with polio.* Boston: Beacon Press.

[58] Lewin, Philip. 1941. *Infantile paralysis: Anterior poliomyelitis.* Philadelphia: W. B. Saunders Company.

[59] Lindell, John Earl and Ethel Brooks Lindell. 1988. *Oh, God, help me! For I cannot help myself: A true story of faith in the life of a polio survivor.* Tempe, AZ: John E. Lindell.

[60] Lippman, Theo, Jr. 1977. *The squire of Warm Springs: F. D. R. in Georgia 1924–1945.* Chicago: Playboy Press.

[61] Longmore, Paul K. 2003. *Why I burned my book and other essays on disability.* Philadelphia: Temple University Press.

[62] Longmore, Paul K., and Lauri Umansky, ed. 2001. *The new disability history: American perspectives.* New York: New York University Press.

[63] Lovering, Robert. 1993. *Out of the darkness: Coping with disability.* Phoenix: Associated Rehabilitation Counseling Specialists.

[64] Marshall, Alan. 1955. *I can jump puddles.* Melbourne: Cheshire.

[65] Martin, Emily. 1994. *Flexible bodies: Tracking immunity in American culture from the days of polio to the age of AIDS.* Boston: Beacon Press.

[66] Marugg, Jim. 1955. *Beyond endurance.* London: Rupert Hart-Davis.

[67] Mason, Martha. 2003. *Breath: Life in the rhythm of an iron lung.* Asheboro, NC : Down Home Press.

[68] Mason, Mary Grimley. 2000. *Life prints: A memoir of healing and discovery.* New York: The Feminist Press.

[69] McPherson, Stephanie Sammartino. 2002. *Jonas Salk: Conquering polio.* Minneapolis: Lerner Publications Co.

[70] Mee, Charles L. 1999. *A nearly normal life: A memoir.* Boston: Little, Brown and Company.

[71] ———1977. *A visit to Haldeman and other states of mind.* New York: M. Evans and Company.

[72] Milam, Lorenzo. 1984. *Cripple liberation front marching band blues*. San Diego: Mho & Mho Works.

[73] ————1993. *Cripzen: A manual for survival*. San Diego: Mho & Mho Works.

[74] Needham, J. B., and R. Taylor. 1959. *Looking up*. New York: Putnam.

[75] O'Brien, Mark. 2003. *How I became a human being: A disabled man's quest for independence*. Madison, WI: University of Wisconsin Press.

[76] Oldstone, Michael B. A. 1998. *Viruses, plagues, & history*. New York: Cambridge University Press.

[77] Opie, June. 1957. *Over my dead body*. London: Methuen.

[78] Oshinsky, David M. 2005. *Polio: An American story*. New York: Oxford University Press.

[79] Paul, John R. 1971. *A history of poliomyelitis*. New Haven: Yale University Press.

[80] Plagemann, B. 1949. *My place to stand*. New York: Farrar, Straus.

[81] Pohl, John F., M. Pohl, and Elizabeth Kenny. 1943. *The Kenny concept of infantile paralysis and its treatment*. Minneapolis: Bruce Publishing Company.

[82] Reynolds, R. J. S. 1956. *Physical measures in the treatment of poliomyelitis*. London: Faber and Faber.

[83] Rogers, Naomi. 1992. *Dirt and disease: Polio before FDR*. New Brunswick, NJ: Rutgers University Press.

[84] Rusk, Howard and Eugene Taylor. 1958. *Rehabilitation medicine*. St. Louis: Mosby.

[85] Salgado, Sebastião. 2001. *The end of polio: A global effort to end a disease*. Boston: Bulfinch Press.

Walking Isn't Everything

[86] Sass, Edmund. J., George Gottfried, and Anthony Sorem. 1996. *Polio's legacy: An oral history.* Lanham, MD: University Press of America.

[87] Saxton, Marsha and Florence Howe, eds. 1987. *With wings: An anthology of literature by and about women with disabilities.* New York: Feminist Press.

[88] Seavey, Nina G., Jane S. Smith, and Paul Wagner. 1998. *A paralyzing fear: Conquering polio in America.* New York: TV Books.

[89] Shapiro, Joseph P. 1993. *No pity: People with disabilities forging a new civil rights movement.* New York: Times Books.

[90] Sheed, Wilfrid. 1995. *In love with daylight: A memoir of recovery.* New York: Simon & Schuster.

[91] Shreve, Susan R. 2007. *Warm Springs: Traces of a childhood at FDR's polio haven.* Boston: Houghton Mifflin.

[92] Sills, David. 1957. *The volunteers: Means and ends in a national organization.* Glencoe, Il: Free Press.

[93] Silver, Julie K. 2001. *Post-Polio syndrome: A guide for polio survivors and their families.* New Haven, CT: Yale University Press.

[94] Silver, Julie K., and Anne C. Gawne. 2004. *Postpolio syndrome.* Philadelphia: Hanley & Belfus.

[95] Sink, Alice E. 1998. *The grit behind the miracle: A true story of the determination and hard work behind an emergency infantile paralysis hospital, 1944–1945.* Lanham, MD: University Press of America.

[96] Smart, Julie. 2001. *Disability, society, and the individual.* Gaithersburg, MD: Aspen Publishers, Inc.

[97] Smith, Jane S. 1990. *Patenting the sun: Polio and the Salk vaccine.* New York: W. Morrow.

[98] Sternburg, Louis and Dorothy Sternburg. 1986. *View from the seesaw.* New York: Dodd, Mead, and Company.

[99] Thomson, Rosemarie Garland. 1997. *Extraordinary bodies: Figuring physical disability in American culture and literature.* New York: Columbia University.

[100] Troan, John. 2000. *Passport to adventure, or, how a typewriter from Santa led to an exciting lifetime journey: A memoir.* Pittsburgh: Neworks Press.

[101] Walker, Turnley. 1950. *Rise up and walk.* New York: Dutton.

[102] ———1953. *Roosevelt and the Warm Springs story.* New York: A. A. Wyn.

[103] Walters, Anne and Jim Marugg. 1954. *Beyond endurance.* New York: Harper.

[104] Ward, John W. and Christian Warren. 2007. *Silent victories: The history and practice of public health in twentieth-century America.* New York: Oxford University Press.

[105] Waterson, A. P. and Lise Wilkinson. 1978. *An introduction to the history of virology.* Cambridge, NY: Cambridge University Press.

[106] Wendell, Susan. 1996. *The rejected body: Feminist philosophical reflections on disability.* New York: Routledge.

[107] Willmuth, Mary E. and Lillian Holcomb, eds. 1994. *Women with disabilities: Found voices.* Binghamton, NY: Haworth Press.

[108] Wilson, Daniel J. 2005. *Living with polio: The epidemic and its survivors.* Chicago: The University of Chicago Press.

[109] Wilson, John Rowan. 1963. *Margin of safety: The story of poliomyeli tis vaccine.* London: Collins.

[110] Winter, Roger. (1971). *I'll walk tomorrow.* Anderson, IN: Warner Press.

[111] Winter, Roger and Kenneth F. Hall. 1964. *Point after touchdown*. Anderson, IN: Warner Press.

[112] Woods, Regina. 1994. *Tales from inside the iron lung (and how I got out of it)*. Philadelphia: University of Pennsylvania Press.

[113] Zames, Frieda and Doris Zames Fleischer. 2001. *The disability rights movement: From charity to confrontation*. Philadelphia: Temple University Press.

[114] Zola, Irving Kenneth. 1982. *Missing pieces: A chronicle of living with a disability*. Philadelphia: Temple University Press.

[115] ———1982. *Ordinary lives: Voices of disability & disease*. Cambridge, MA: Applewood Books.

[116] ———1983. *Socio-medical inquiries: Recollections, reflections, and reconsiderations*. Philadelphia: Temple University Press.

About the Author

Jean Lucille Leeper was born in Akron, Ohio on October 23, 1917, the only child of Nellie J. Hine and Henry Lloyd Leeper. Her mother was a registered nurse and her father a streetcar conductor and machinist. Jean attended public school and graduated from Buchtel High School in Akron in 1935. She had not settled on a career when she graduated. She was ambitious and pretty and harbored a fantasy of a singing/stage career. However, her voice was mediocre at best and Akron not the place from which to launch a stage career. She enrolled in nursing school at Akron City Hospital but quit after one semester. She was independent and lacked the discipline to apply herself to subjects that did not interest her. She loved animals, dogs particularly, but saw no career opportunities for a young woman in the veterinary field in those days. She hoped a move to a larger city would provide a direction for her ambitions.

In 1940, she moved to Detroit to see what a larger city actually had to offer. She found a job as a hostess at Stouffer's restaurant in downtown Detroit and roomed with family friends. A mutual friend introduced her to Harry Denecke later that year. Harry was a good looking, affable, but serious young man working as a salesman for U.S. Printing and Lithograph Co. Also working in the Detroit office of U.S. Printing and Lithograph was Harry's father, Ferd Denecke, and his brother, Robert Denecke. U.S. Printing specialized in print advertising for major companies, including the automobile companies headquartered in Detroit. Harry had received his degree in business from Western Michigan Teachers College in 1939 and Jean considered him a good catch. They dated steadily and when Harry was drafted in 1941, Jean was disappointed he had not presented her with an engagement ring.

After he completed basic training later in 1941, Harry invited Jean to visit him in Leesville, Louisiana where he was temporarily stationed. She often said that her attempts to convince him the war would not interfere with their happiness were ignored. Harry did not think it was a good time to get married. However, the night before she was supposed to leave to return to Detroit, Harry failed to make their connection and did not catch up to her until very late in the evening. As he searched the small town for her, he feared she had returned to Detroit without saying goodbye. They were married the next day in Leesville.

Jean and Harry made a good team. They were very much in love and their personalities were complementary. She was driving and ambitious and he was levelheaded and easygoing. Harry headed to Officers Candidate School (OCS) at Camp Beale, California, near Marysville, and Jean accompanied him. They enjoyed traveling in California and Nevada before Harry was shipped overseas in 1943 after completing OCS. During this time, Jean bought her beloved cocker spaniel, Mandy, in 1942, and their daughter, Kristin, was born in Yuba City, California in late 1943. Harry was commissioned a second lieutenant and served with distinction in the 13th Armored Division in France and Germany. The "Black Cat" Division, as the 13th was known, was trained at Camp Beale, California and Camp Bowie, Texas during 1942 and 1943. They were deployed from Le Havre, France in January 1945 and moved across France liberating towns until

March 25 when they crossed the German border. The division performed cleanup operations as it advanced toward the Rhine. By April 1945, they had liberated the towns of Zweibrucken, Overstein, Frankfurt, Limburg, Aschaefenburg, Bamberg, Erlangen, Nurnberg and others as they drove toward Austria. In May of 1945, operations were halted and the European war ended. Harry received the Bronze Star for valor after leading a dangerous reconnaissance mission that successfully surprised the enemy and rescued his platoon.

By the time Harry went overseas, Jean's parents had moved to Detroit when her father's job with Whitman Barnes relocated there. Jean and Kris lived with Jean's parents until Harry was discharged in 1945.

When the war was over, Jean and Harry bought a home in Dearborn Heights, Michigan that Jean had been able to find right before the war ended. Although the house was small and hastily built, they were lucky to find affordable and available housing during that period of severe housing shortages. Harry went back to his job at U.S. Printing and Lithograph and they began a stable life together for the first time since their marriage.

In the fall of 1947, Jean contracted polio after a vacation trip to northern Michigan. She spent nine months, from September 1947 to May 1948, in Herman Kiefer Hospital in Detroit. Polio care was primitive in those days; Jean experienced many frustrating and painful treatments in Herman Kiefer that tested her will to live. She was also dismayed to find that several close friends were unnecessarily afraid of exposure to polio by being in her presence, months after there was no danger of contagion. This physical and social isolation was difficult for her. She missed her dog, missed her daughter, missed her friends, and missed having a normal life. Harry and her parents visited often during this hospital stay and shored up her will to live.

Finally, after nine months, she was able to return home in an iron lung to assist her breathing. Her immediate goal was to breathe without the aid of the iron lung, which she accomplished in a matter of months. Her family spent the next year adjusting to the schedule of caring for a person with polio and trying various combinations of nursing and home care for Jean while Harry worked and Kris began school. Her mother and father were a tremendous help to her during this process and could always be counted on to care for Kris and run errands. After much trial and error, Harry and Jean found a dependable weekday housekeeper and a more normal routine was established that the family more or less followed for the rest of Jean's life.

From October 1948 until the end of February 1949, Jean was a patient at the Roosevelt Foundation in Warms Springs, Georgia. Warm Springs, founded and endowed by Franklin Roosevelt and bequeathed to the State of Georgia after his death, had an international reputation for progressive polio treatment. Although apprehensive at first, Jean received care that would teach her techniques she was able to use to improve her functioning for the rest of her life. She was fitted with braces and a proper wheelchair and underwent a comprehensive routine of physical therapy and rehabilitation. There she learned to feed and groom herself, dial a telephone, write, even do needlework. The doctors were honest with her and told her there was no part of her body that polio had not affected. She never regained the ability to walk and was always dependent upon others to transfer her to her wheelchair and dress her. However, with a lapboard that attached to her wheelchair like a small table, she was able to have whatever she needed brought to her and work from that small board. Her arms were supported by cuffs at the wrist and elbow and suspended from springs that ran on steel rods above her wheelchair. The rods were attached to the wheelchair and could be easily removed when not in use. This set-up allowed Jean to swing and move her arms, giving her the necessary arm mobility to manage many everyday tasks. She returned from Warm Springs with new friends, new hope, and a determination to live as full and independent a life as possible.

Upon her return from Warm Springs in 1949, Jean became active in her church, Girl Scouts, and the March of Dimes. She did her work on the telephone and put her organizational skills to good use in persuading others to get involved in causes for which she was working. She ran her household as well. She selected the family menus, bought clothes for her daughter and herself over the telephone, helped with homework, and supervised the household help five days a week. Harry and Kris shared care duties on the weekend, and Jean supervised them as well.

Jean also began working on this book during those years. She enlisted her friend, and professional secretary, Betty Isom, to assist her. Betty came to Jean's house in her free time and as Jean dictated, Betty recorded a rough draft. Jean and Betty then went over each draft until they were satisfied with the wording. Jean's intention was to provide a book to inspire other people with polio to work not only toward recovery but to live a full life with whatever disabilities remained. Jean and Betty worked on the book for a little over a year. When it was finished, Jean sent it to several publishers. Most submissions were politely declined, but a few suggested revisions. Those revisions were never made, probably because Jean became so busy with a new endeavor she could not find the time.

In 1952, the family moved to the home of Jean's parents in Dearborn, Michigan after Jean's mother died and her father remarried. Jean felt she needed a bigger challenge and one night, she saw on television the story of a person who had started a babysitters registry from her home. Jean felt it was something she could do from her wheelchair. She researched the business possibilities extensively and in 1954 founded Rock-A-Bye Sitters Registry, starting with a few friends and women from her church.

The business was confined to her city of residence, Dearborn, Michigan and showed a small profit after only a few months. Its customers, who were for the most part families with an active social life, were happy to pay a small premium for a reliable adult babysitter of their choice and have the details reliably arranged and confirmed for them. Although the business remained small out of necessity, Jean was proud of her financial contribution to the family. The cost of employing household help five days a week was high, particularly in those days before Social Security Disability. Jean ran the business and it continued to prosper until Jean's death in 1969.

Jean and Harry began to take short trips to see if they could manage travel. Harry had purchased a VW bus as the family car because of the ease of lifting Jean out of her wheelchair and into the bus, which was configured much like a modern day van. He found he did not need to bend over to slide her into the car seat, thus making the transfer much easier on his back. The bus also provided sufficient and convenient storage for Jean's wheelchair and other necessities of life with polio such as her lapboard and arm slings. Although most of their socializing was done at their home, Jean and Harry were able to attend family celebrations and special occasions such as weddings, graduation ceremonies, and even art exhibits and museums.

Their first extended trip was to Akron, Ohio to visit Jean's close childhood friend, Marguerite Myers and her husband. The trip went well and Jean and Harry were encouraged to venture farther, their favorite destination being Williamsburg, Virginia and the surrounding area.

With assistance, and particularly support from her husband, she raised her family, ran her household, and was an inspiration to others. Jean retained her independent attitude, but she needed support in virtually every aspect of daily living. She needed to have everything she used brought to her and then taken away when she was finished. Harry put Jean in her wheelchair in the morning before he left for work, and her housekeeper put Jean back into bed, with the help of a hydraulic lift, around noon. She ran her business from her bed the rest of the day until Harry came home from work, returned her to her wheelchair for dinner, and put her back to bed at night. In the evening, Harry often worked in his darkroom or built model trains. Jean worked on needlework, researched recipes, or played cards with Kris.

The reliable employment of housekeeper Della Pelmore blossomed into a friendship that survived nearly twenty years of a compatible working relationship. Her contributions and support to the family cannot be overstated. Miss Pelmore helped raise Kris and was Jean's eyes and ears both in the house and around the neighborhood. Miss Pelmore began cooking each night's meal and Harry finished it when he arrived home from work.

The weekend schedule was a bit more relaxed, but Jean's routine remained much the same. Harry did the grocery shopping on Saturday morning while Kris was available to support Jean in the home. Saturday evenings were usually spent playing bridge with friends.

Kris had always been encouraged to be independent. Her life was the typical one of friends, school, and social events. Kris and her mother suffered through the usual mother/daughter trauma of the teenage years. Jean was supportive of Kris, but made it clear she expected Kris to not only work part-time while in high school, but go to college, too. Jean spent many hours with Kris reviewing college catalogues and exploring various career opportunities. Jean's attitude about the potential of women was ahead of her time. She taught Kris to value financial independence and to plan to support herself.

As Jean and Harry grew older, Jean expressed some anxiety about what might happen to her if Harry died or if he became disabled. The family did not deal with the issue openly.

There seemed to be no satisfactory answer, so life continued as always, with everyone hoping for the best.

Harry's support throughout the years was steadfast and astounding to many who knew Jean and him. More than one woman confessed to Jean that she wondered if her own husband would stand by her under similar circumstances. If Jean thought Harry capable of less, she never told anyone, and when asked by a friend if she had led a happy life, she answered, "yes."

Jean lived to see Kris graduate from college, marry, and have her career as a social worker with the State of Michigan. Jean Denecke died in her sleep of a cerebral hemorrhage March 10, 1969 at her home in Dearborn, Michigan.

Jean's death stunned Harry and Kris, as well as her friends, family, and customers of Rock-A-Bye Sitters Registry. Jean's funeral was well attended, with many people remarking on her active and courageous life. Less well received by Harry and Kris were those comments by others who suggested they might be relieved by not having to care for Jean anymore.

In fact, Harry and Kris suddenly had a huge gap in their lives. They had lost a spouse and mother they loved, but they had also lost the sense that someone had really needed them in a special and all encompassing way. Kris no longer lived at home, but she had been in daily contact with her mother and relied on her support and friendship. Harry's challenges were a bit more complicated.

For the first time in many years, Harry had time on his hands and he did not know how to fill it. He considered a career change, even considered studying law, but he had many years in at U.S. Printing and Lithograph and felt he needed to continue building his pension. He was fifty-two years old and not ready to retire, nor was he, realistically, ready to start again from scratch. Harry traveled as much as he was able, often stopping to visit

Jean's lifetime friend, Marguerite Myers, in Akron on the way to the Smokies. Alaska was also a favorite destination.

Kris, who had been divorced in 1968, and Harry spent a lot of time together the first year after Jean's death. They grieved together, faced up to returning to restaurants they had enjoyed as a family, and discussed future plans. In October 1969, Harry took Kris on a trip to California by train. They visited the place of her birth, the kennel where the family dog was bred and born, drove by Kris' first house in Marysville, ate at wonderful restaurants, and stayed at the best hotels, once with the manager apologizing to Harry for not giving them adjoining rooms. Because of the name difference, many hoteliers assumed Harry was traveling with a young woman who was not his wife. Harry told Kris he liked traveling with her because that very assumption also got him the best accommodations and the best service at restaurants when they were together. Kris never forgot that wonderful trip and always smiled at the memory of their being mistaken for an older man with his young girlfriend. How could anyone miss the family resemblance?

During that time, Harry began seeing more of a family friend, Dawn Burroughs. Dawn and her former husband had known Harry and Jean while they were in the service and the friendship continued over the years. Dawn was the mother of two grown children, Doug and Barbara. Jean and Dawn had been good friends over the years, with Dawn having been a frequent bridge partner of Jean's. Dawn and Harry had suffered a mutual loss and found themselves natural companions, which grew into a more serious relationship as time went on.

In February of 1972, Kris called Harry to tell him she had decided to remarry. During this happy conversation, Kris teasingly asked Harry when he was going to marry Dawn. He had no immediate response, but three weeks later, Harry phoned Kris and said, "I think I will." Kris, involved in wedding plans and not thinking about their earlier conversation, inquired as to what it was he thought he would do. Harry said he was going to marry Dawn. Kris was delighted. She had always been fond of Dawn and knew her father needed love and companionship. Dawn and Harry seemed right for each other. Kris was teasing her dad about getting married because he had been able to get his "old maid" daughter married off when the conversation suddenly took a serious turn. Harry said, "You don't think lightning would strike twice in the same place, do you?" Kris acknowledged Harry's concern as they discussed the situation, with Harry explaining to Kris that he had built model trains in the evening as a way to entertain himself and still be at home and available to Jean. Kris had always thought he had built them because he was a train buff. It had not fully occurred to her that this activity was Harry's occupational therapy and a way to forget his responsibilities for a time. Kris reassured him that he should "just get married and be happy." Their conversation lingered always in Kris' mind as the only time in her memory that her father had expressed the toll Jean's polio had taken on him.

Harry and Dawn married in May 1972 in Dearborn, Michigan. They sold Dawn's condominium and looked for a house but ultimately decided to remodel and redecorate Harry's home in Dearborn. It was a practical decision. Dawn was about to retire from Chrysler Corporation, where she had been an executive secretary, and Harry was not sure of the future of his job.

U.S. Printing and Lithograph had merged and expanded several times, ultimately becoming Diamond International Corporation. In 1975, Harry was offered a buyout. He took it and landed a job the next day with a printing company headquartered in Cleveland, Ohio. The agreement was that Harry would work from his home and attend a sales meeting in Cleveland once a month. Harry was hired for his contacts with the auto industry and was well compensated for his experience and knowledge.

Harry and Dawn continued to travel and entertain friends and family at home. Kris enjoyed the holiday company of Dawn's children who both lived busy and active lives in other states.

In late 1985, Harry went to his doctor, complaining of fatigue. He had had earlier heart bypass surgery and thought his problem had returned. Tests showed he had leukemia. Harry received non-aggressive treatment and seemed to be doing well. He and Dawn traveled to New Orleans but returned early because Harry, who had never lost a day's work to illness, came down with a serious respiratory infection. He recovered, but on July 13, 1986, Harry was rushed to Oakwood Hospital with pneumonia. He was admitted and died shortly after that from an acute leukemic blast. Kris did not make it to the hospital in time to say goodbye to her father. Harry Denecke was sixty-nine years old.

Jean wrote this book to provide encouragement to others. It is uniquely her story but also the story of a family of ordinary people living ordinary lives. There are no heroes in this book. This family laughed, cried, and squabbled like all others. It faced everyday petty annoyances and larger crises and somehow coped and found solutions. Kris believes they were, often, just plain lucky.

Kristin Gruenewald and Keith Storey

Did you like this book?

If you enjoyed this book, you will find more interesting books at
www.CrystalDreamsPublishing.com

Please take the time to let us know how you liked this book. Even short reviews of 2-3 sentences can be helpful and may be used in our marketing materials. If you take the time to post a review for this book on Amazon.com, let us know when the review is posted and you will receive a free audiobook or ebook from our catalog. Simply email the link to the review once it is live on Amazon.com, your name, and your mailing address -- send the email to orders@mmpubs.com with the subject line "Book Review Posted on Amazon."

If you have questions about this book, our customer loyalty program, or our review rewards program, please contact us at info@mmpubs.com.

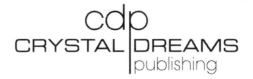

a division of Multi-Media Publications Inc.

CPSIA information can be obtained at www.ICGtesting.com
Printed in the USA
LVOW130555060712

288826LV00002B/88/P